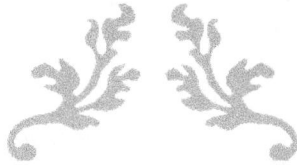

THE HEALING
POWER OF RUNNING

A Guide to Healing the Body, Mind, and Spirit

Jennifer Bonn

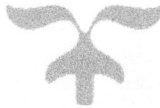

Loving Healing Press

Ann Arbor, MI

The Healing Power of Running: A Guide to Healing the Body, Mind, and Spirit

ISBN 978-1-61599-796-1   paperback
ISBN 978-1-61599-797-8   hardcover
ISBN 978-1-61599-798-5   eBook

Published by
Loving Healing Press   info@LHPress.com
5145 Pontiac Trail   www.LHPress.com
Ann Arbor, MI 48105   Tollfree 888-761-6268

Distributed by Ingram Book Group (USA, CAN, EU, AU) and New Leaf (USA)

Contents

What People Are Saying About
The Healing Power of Running

"*The Healing Power of Running* is a book of realistic and actual events that can occur in anyone's life at any given point. It explains ways that running has helped others strive and be successful in healing, whether it is physically or mentally. I found myself laughing, crying and thinking, "Hmm... I need to do this!" It's empowering and makes you want to RUN like there is no tomorrow. The best part is it makes you want to create a bond with strangers, who become family. Read the book, and you, too, will want to heal by running."

Kim Turner,
Aircraft mechanic III-gen-mods

"Jennifer Bonn writes an extremely helpful, energetic and thera-peutic book on the challenges and rewards of running. The stories and examples, shared by the runners – with perfect notes about their journeys –will help both beginners and seasoned runners; Bonn's own running experiences alone are worth the read. She finds easy ways to explain how running can become addictive and life changing. I'll become a healthier person, and possibly a better runner, just by reading it. The tips, guidance and instructions are what most of us could use in life, and it can be applied anywhere."

Hal Cottingham,
Director of operations, Global Technology Services

"*The Healing Power of Running* is a very educational and enjoyable read. Through the anecdotes of friends and experts, Bonn threads the power of running throughout the text. Her love of running is palpable, making me want to pick up running myself. This is an inspirational book that will motivate any reader to be the best version of him/herself and informs beginners the things they need to jumpstart running in a safe manner. Anyone who runs, or wants to start, will find something to enjoy about this book."

Lucy Kirby,
Librarian

"Does life exhaust you? Has your body let you down, one way or another, including life-threatening conditions like MS or cancer? Are you addicted to food or nasty drugs or maybe miserable and full of anxiety? This little book by Jennifer Bonn will inspire you to climb out of your hole by running. For most of my life, I have found running to be a positive addiction, and it has benefited me in many of the ways Jen describes. If you want to transform your life, you can't do too much better than allow *The Healing Power of Running* to inspire you."

Bob Rich, PhD, author of *From Depression to Contentment*

1 Why I Run

When I think of what running means to me, the first word that comes to mind is healing. Running has been like a good friend who knows exactly what you need when times are hard, is there without judging, and who loves to see you grow. Running has saved me physically and mentally throughout my life. It is responsible for my sanity and for keeping me thriving without any medications. It has strengthened me and allowed me to push myself to the limits. It has also introduced me to an amazing running community that has supported me and taught me many important lessons. Let me tell you about my running journey.

I went to schools in New England that required all students to do three seasons of sports activities, so being active was nothing new, but I looked at running as something we did for conditioning. If you had asked me to go for a run for fun, I would have thought you were crazy. Now, my neighbors think I'm the crazy one because I'm running in the neighborhood every day in all sorts of weather.

During my senior year in college, I noticed that my love of food was adding some pounds to my waistline, so I began to run with some friends. We had fun running around campus and talking about everything. It was the first time I was running for fun, and I realized I enjoyed my runs.

My first job as a teacher was at a boarding school, and one of my duties was to coach. I decided if I was going to ask my athletes to be in good shape, I had to be in good condition as well. I began running regularly. Any teacher will tell you the first year is tough, so I started to use my runs as my escape. I could run away from a bad day or use it to have some quiet time. During forty years of teaching, running continued to be a form of stress relief as well as a way to leave the conflict and noise behind me. Any time I needed to relax, I went for a long run.

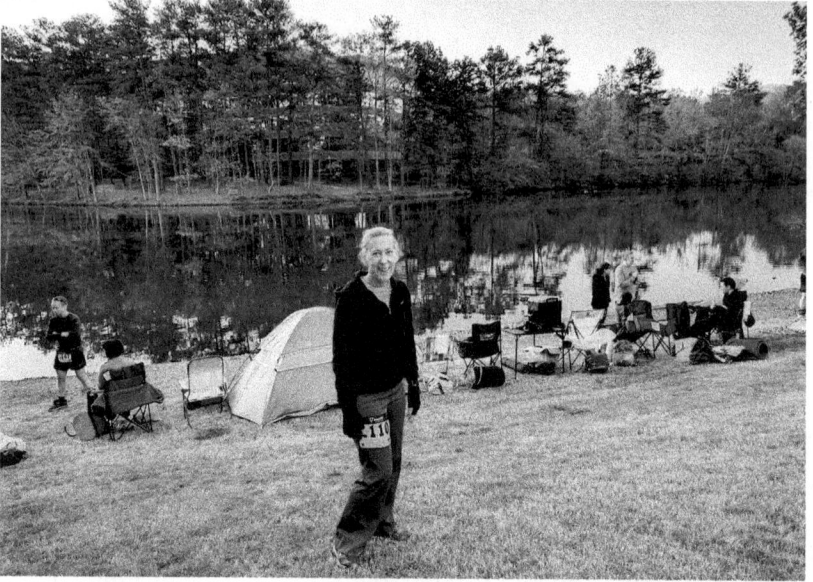

My first ultra was a 27-mile learning experience

I had no idea how much of a lifesaver it would be until my son was born. He started having seizures, and tests showed he had a leaking blood vessel in his brain. We were told our choice was to operate on his brain with a fifty percent chance of survival, or not operate with the risk he would be impaired mentally. We chose the operation, and thankfully he survived. He had a huge lump on the side of his head for several months, and although it shouldn't have bothered me, there was a lot of pity about the situation from others. They assumed he would be mentally impaired without even asking. Five days after giving birth, I laced up my sneakers and went for a long run. I was overwhelmed by every emotion you could imagine and running gave me a chance to escape. During this time, running kept me sane.

Running saved me again when my husband battled an addiction to alcohol. I was pregnant with our third child, and once again, I felt like life was overwhelming me, so I turned to my constant friend, and I ran it out.

This continued to be a pattern anytime I was overwhelmed. Running was something I could control when everything else in my life was chaos. I cannot imagine having to cope without the outlet running gives me. As I started to go to races, I began to hear other people with similar stories to mine. I heard the different ways running has been a Godsend in different situations.

Running helped me socially as well. I met my best friends through running, and they have been my support for many years. I may never have met them if it had not been for running. Everyone needs their tribe, and my running friends are mine. I don't know if it is the feel-good endorphins that running produces, but runners are the nicest people.

I became the cross-country coach at one school where I taught. I wanted to teach the runners that running could be fun, so I incorporated running games into our training. I wanted them to fall in love with running. Not only did they fall in love with the sport, but they also learned how running could bring people together. We had several runners who had not been successful in other sports, but they were loved and supported on our team. Even if they came in last, the rest of the team would be screaming and cheering as they crossed the line. Runners would stay after practice and ask if we could jog the trail and talk. I listened to what was happening in their lives, what they were struggling with, and what advice they needed. It was a group of runners sharing our lives and getting stronger at the same time. We were helping each other with both our mental and physical health.

The first race I ever ran was called The Josh Billings Race. It was a relay race where one person did the 6-mile run, one person biked 18 miles, and two people canoed a two-mile loop. I was so nervous, and I kept asking myself, "Do they know this is my first race?" I didn't want to let them down. That first 10 k ended up being my personal best for my whole life. I also discovered that the rest of my team was more worried about the beer and food after the race than about how well they did.

My husband ran a marathon (26.2 miles) before I did. A group of friends at work convinced him to join them, and the training began. They kept each other accountable, and the training was very intense. I was worried at one point because John had lost so much weight because he was running so many miles. They ran in weather that most people would not want to be out in. It didn't matter if it was snowing, sleeting, whether there was ice, or what the temperature was. They were out running, pushing each other to the limits. The marathon experience for John was about the camaraderie and the support he and his friends gave each other more than it was about the miles he ran.

A run like a marathon is often a unique experience with more than one memorable story to tell at the end. My first one was the Atlanta marathon, and I remember being happy to have the opportunity to finally run the distance. The Atlanta course had the most hills of any marathon I have done. As I was walking up one of the bigger hills, the man next to me said, "Are you using the Jeff Galloway method?" (Jeff Galloway is an elite runner who believes walking is a great way to run longer.) I replied, "I'm using the I'm trying to survive method."

My favorite distance is the ultramarathon, which is anything farther than 26.2 miles. One of my friends once asked me, "Do you think you will ever do an ultra?" I replied, "Absolutely not!" I could not imagine running longer than 26.2 miles, which proves that the impossible becomes possible when you do it. I learned so much about my body and how to protect it. I learned how to fight nausea, protect my feet, fuel, and hydrate, and I learned how resilient the body can be if you let it rest for a bit. Ultras taught me that almost anything is possible, and it introduced me to people who refuse to let life get them down. When they are faced with a roadblock, they find a way around it. Being around people like that not only inspires you but also heals you because you see the strong spirit that people have.

Here is more of a description of what benefits running gives to me.

Weight management

This is of course the reason many people run. Runners need calories to fuel their running, which means you might be able to eat more than non-runners. I started running because I love good food, but I wanted to be able to stay at a reasonable weight. While running helped me in this aspect, it also opened up the other possibilities running can offer.

Self-esteem

For most of my life, I have struggled with the feeling that I'm not good enough, that I'm somehow less than I should be. I discovered I was good at running. I could set goals and find ways to become better. No one criticized how I was doing it, because there are so many ways to achieve the goals. It gave me the confidence I lacked.

Quiet time

As a teacher and a mother, I am surrounded by noise all the time. Running gives me the quiet time I need to recharge. When I'm running, I can work out problems and be creative, or I can let my mind rest while I enjoy the beauty around me.

Therapy

Running can provide mental health benefits. Running can be used as therapy because whenever my world was crashing down around me, I could go for a long run and run off whatever emotion was holding me back. I have never turned to substances for relief; it has always been running that helps me through difficult periods.

Physical

Running has kept me in excellent health throughout the years. At sixty-three, I am not on any medications, which always perplexes the urgent care providers. Once, when I had to go to urgent care because I had burst stitches on my arm with the last punch in Karate class, the nurse told me that the blood pressure machine must not be working and said the same thing when she took my pulse because both were so low. Running allows me to keep pushing my limits and becoming stronger.

Social

I discovered quickly that races are social events. I have met some of my best friends through running. It has become a very important community to me.

Scott Jurek describes his passion for running in his book, *Eat and Run*. "Running is what I do. Running is what I love. Running is to a large extent who I am. In the sport I have chosen as an avocation, career obsession, and unerring but merciless teacher, running is how I answer any challenge. I ran because overcoming the difficulties of an ultramarathon reminded me that I could overcome the difficulties of life, that overcoming was life." (pp. 2 and 6)

I love that Scott describes running as a teacher because I agree with him 100%. Running can teach you that the impossible is possible, that you can push beyond limits, you can do crazy, epic, memorable things, meet people who will change your life, and most of all, you can learn how to be the best version of yourself.

I hope you will enjoy it as I share the stories of some of the ways running has healed others in powerful ways.

2   Running for Recovery

I signed up for a race several years ago, called "Run for Recovery," without thinking much about the name, and I had no idea I would hear so many stories there. Several of the runners shared with me how running has saved their lives as they struggled with addiction. I will always remember one man who said to me, "I would not be here talking to you right now if I had not started running." We headed back again this year and as we were standing around after the race the announcer asked, "How many of you have fought addiction?" Many hands went up. He then asked, "How many of you have had a friend or family member who has been an addict?" Almost every hand went up. The announcer also mentioned that the number of people at the race had doubled from the year before, so more people were seeing the benefit of running to heal them. So, what is it about running and exercise that can help with addiction?

Running is a healthy outlet. It's a coping strategy for addiction, and a healthy way to manage stress, and calm your mind, and overcome depression and anxiety.

In her article, "Six Benefits of Exercise and Addiction Recovery," Nicole LaNeve says that once substances are removed, the addict may be anxious or depressed, and physical activity can help with negative emotions. Running can improve mood, reduce stress, and help with sleep. Recovery can leave you tired, and exercise can give you energy. Regular movement has been proven to prevent people from returning to alcohol or drug use.

On the website, www.podiumrunner.com, in the article, "Why Running is Good for Addiction Recovery," Candice Rasa lists the following ways that running can help:

- A strong sense of positive feelings
- Reduced depression
- Reduced craving for unhealthy food and drugs

- Increased sense of being in control
- Clearer thinking
- Higher sense of achievement
- Greater hope for future

"How Exercise Can Help With Addiction Recovery," written by Keri Wiginton says that exercise and drugs work on similar parts of the brain. They both activate your reward pathway which triggers feel-good chemicals like Serotonin and Dopamine.

Running can build a social network that can support anyone including a recovering addict. Runners tend to be very encouraging and supportive. There are always stories of inspiration and grit within this community.

My friend, Sally, says running helped her to stop smoking. She says running has been the constant in her life for thirty-five years. It is always there to help her make it through a rough spot. Her struggles with anxiety could have led her to look for relief through alcohol or harmful drugs, but running gave her the calming effects she needed.

Dr. Nora Volkow, director of The National Institute on Drug Abuse in the U.S., says, "The studies are showing that there's an effect in the interaction between physical activity and the way we respond to drugs." Her thoughts can be read in The Associated Press' article "Working Out May Help Prevent Substance Abuse" (Volkow 2008).

Dr. John Ratey, an associate clinical professor of psychiatry at Harvard Medical School in Boston, says, "When you run, you get a boost in dopamine, noradrenaline, and serotonin, just as if you were taking a little Prozac and Ritalin."

Texas A &M University hosts a yearly run for recovery with the motto "One step at a time." A tab on the campus website, https://studentlife.tamu.edu/hp/run-for-recovery/, explains how running can aid recovery. Here is what it says: "Recovering from addiction is more than just removing alcohol or other drugs from one's life. It's an ongoing process that involves healing on all levels. Footprints Beachside Recovery Center has described unique ways the Eight Dimensions of Wellness apply to those in recovery, listed below:

- **Emotional:** To a large extent, your emotional well-being depends on your willingness and dedication to practice the healthy coping skills you learned in your addiction rehab program. This is also an essential component of relapse prevention.

- **Physical:** Exercise is a great way to repair the damage of long-term drug or alcohol abuse and triggers a natural release of dopamine in the brain's reward center.

- **Spiritual:** Sometimes life is tough. Your spirituality could give you a sense of purpose that may make it easier to cope with difficult situations.

- **Occupational:** If you find satisfaction in your job, consider yourself lucky. People like you often believe their lives feel more rewarding and fulfilling. Not so lucky? Think about volunteering in your community— either by donating your time to those in need or by offering your unique skill set to make life better for the people around you.

- **Intellectual:** Pursuing activities you find interesting is a great way to keep your brain active and to help restore the damage caused by habitual drug or alcohol use.

- **Environmental:** Do what you can to make your living arrangements as pleasant and as stimulating as possible, because your physical environment plays a huge role in your wellbeing.

- **Social:** Social isolation is one of the most common addiction relapse triggers. If you aren't comfortable meeting new people—and some people aren't—try to maintain contact with the friends or family you already have.

- **Financial:** Our finances are a huge source of stress and anxiety, and, unfortunately, we can't make it go away overnight. However, the key to feeling more financially secure is to take small steps each day. This can help you stay in control while you chip away at your debt."

There are many forms of addiction including food addiction, and there are many needs for recovery such as this journey Carl detailed here:

> In 2017 I was 350lbs and started to hike. I enjoyed it and loved being out in nature. I also enjoyed the physical challenge. As I began to hike with others, it became abundantly clear I was in bad shape. I wanted so badly to keep up, and not be the one to slow the group down.
>
> In January 2020, I got the Garmin Fenix 5 as another hiking gadget I didn't need. After wearing it for a week, it told me my VO^2 max was 27 and I was in the physical shape of a 65-year-old (I was 37). I was saddened but not shocked. I decided I would try to run a mile without stopping. I did and came in at a 12:00-minute pace. I felt like I was going to die. I repeated it 2 days later. I was now on my journey. A few months later I was trying to break 30:00 5k and did so in July of that year.
>
> By Thanksgiving, I ran my first half marathon and was down to 260 lbs. All the while, hiking better and feeling fantastic. I began to take my runs to the trails in December of that year. I ran my first trail half marathon in July 2021 and another one in September. I came in under three hours for both races. I ran the NYC marathon in 2021 at 4:29.
>
> I have lost 114lbs running and it has transformed my life. This year I have a full slate of races on my calendar from the breakneck marathon, Virgil crest 50 miler, and the Whiteface Mountain climb. The future is so bright, and I owe a lot of it to running."

One of the things I love about the running community is the support they give others. I have watched crowds run toward the finish line to cheer in the last runner to cross the line, or to applaud those runners who run despite struggles. It is the place to be if you want your spirits lifted.

Back on my feet (BOMF) uses running to help the homeless realize their power to achieve change. They operate running teams in eleven cities across the country. 82% report their health is good or excellent, and 94% describe themselves as hopeful about their futures. 46% of BOMF runners have obtained employment, housing, or both. The website describes the benefits like this. "As participants offer fellowship, mutual encouragement, and account-ability, BOMF makes it possible for people who have experienced terrible things, including great isolation, to socialize and reconnect with others. Participants build or rebuild key aspects of their identities: as athletes, teammates, morning people, or just plain survivors. At the same time, nonresident runners can connect in a meaningful and immediately rewarding way with people with whom they might otherwise never be engaged."

In "How Running Heals the Mind, Body, and Soul," Sarah Marandi-Steves says:

> "Running was my true saving grace. Despite the physical and mental demands, I truly feel as though running healed my soul. Part of my healing journey included nature and music. I find being outside to be so incredibly peaceful and relaxing and music can truly be so healing as losing yourself in music helps quiet the mind. Running allows me to incorporate both. There is no greater feeling than being outside, listening to music, and moving your body simultaneously.
>
> Whenever I am feeling stressed or overwhelmed, I go for a run. Whenever I want to ensure I start my day off on a positive note, I go for a run. Whenever I want to spend time with my friends while also doing something positive and healthy, we go for a run. Whenever I have a lot on my mind and feel my thoughts racing, I go for a run. Whenever I want to clear my head, I go for a run. If it's a beautiful day and I want to be outside, I go for a run. Running is a form of therapy for me. I zone out and focus on one step at a time, one breath at a time, one movement at a time. When else in life are we able to be so present and mindful? For me, it's when I am running. I don't think about anything else other than what I am doing in that moment and for me, it's incredibly healing."

Kathy is a woman I met at my last ultra. She is one of those people who is full of joy, and who can talk a mile a minute. She told me she had been obsessed with running to the point where it was taking most of her time and was her biggest priority. One day, she was in a car accident that almost killed her. The injuries were horrific, and the doctors were not sure if she would be able to walk again. She told me she thinks she had the accident because God wanted her to straighten out her priorities, but she was determined to also run again. It was a tough time recovering, but now she appreciates every step she runs.

Kathy's story is a good example of the grit that runners have. She could have used her injuries as a reason to never run again, but she was determined to fight her way back. She is one of those people I would describe as fearless. As she was talking with me she described the last race she had done in the North Georgia Mountains. She was at the top of the trail when she realized there was a bear in the woods. She said she made her best time ever because she went down that trail so quickly. She has signed up to do the run again. One encounter with a bear would be enough for me.

My friend, Raleigh, is my running husband. He isn't my husband, but we always race together, and everyone thinks we are married. He has had some severe health issues, but he keeps on running. He has had two strokes, a hole in his heart, a heart operation, and sleep issues. After the first stroke, the doctor told him the stroke should have killed him, but his fitness level saved him. The doctor said that according to his vital signs, he could be classified as an elite athlete. Running saved his life. Whenever Raleigh has health issues he says, "This is only temporary. It's not going to defeat me. I have to recover and then I'll be running again." Most runners have the same type of grit. I know I want to be surrounded by that attitude, and I hope some of it will rub off on me.

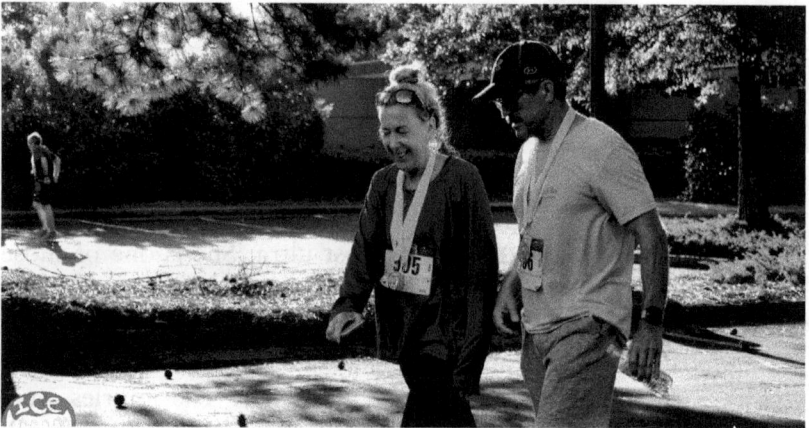

Raleigh and I discussing the race.

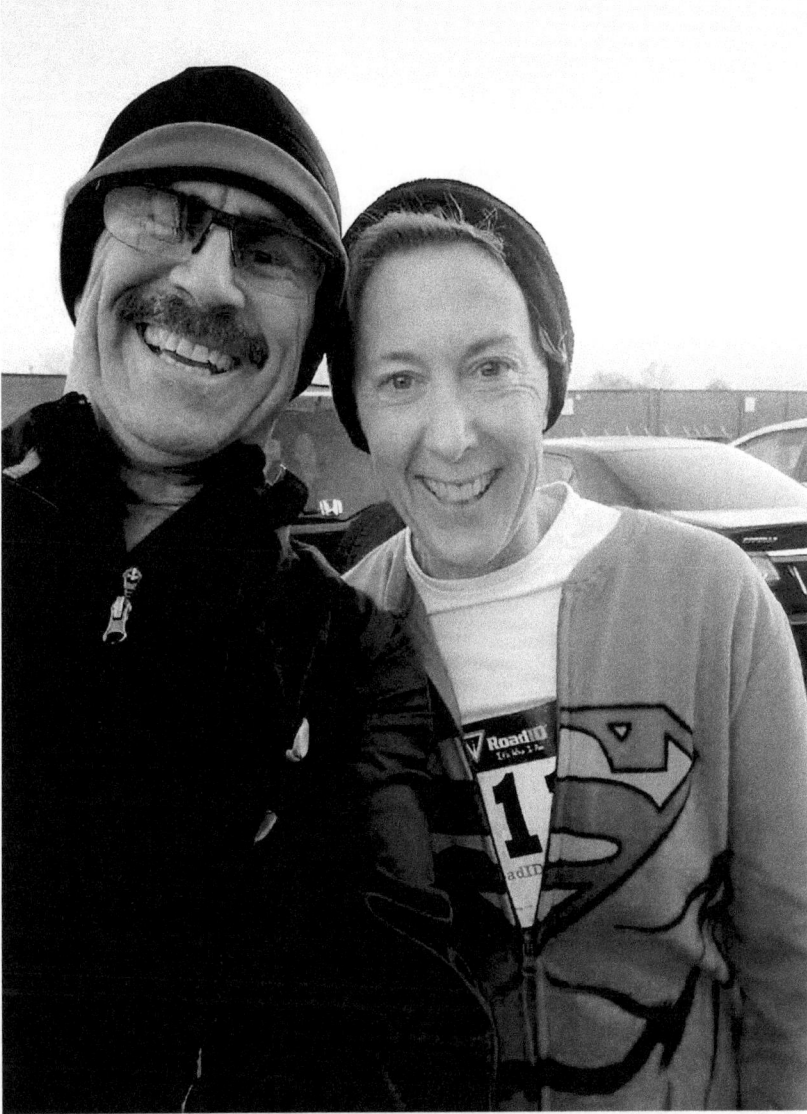

Raleigh and I at the Superman 5K

Raleigh's attitude always inspires me. Most people would be sidelined with the health challenges he has had, but he does the best he can and carries on without any complaining. It makes you realize how important it is for us to be grateful for what we have.

3   Running to Overcome

There is a great movie about overcoming and running called *Overcomer* (2019). Each character in the movie needs to overcome something. A coach loses his football team because the town factory closes, and he is asked to coach cross-country. He only has one runner, who needs healing badly. I love that each member of the coach's family thinks there is nothing to running until they run the course, finish much later than they should, and say, "Why would anyone do that?" Running heals his family, as well as the runner and her family. It is a wonderful story.

Overcomers are faced with huge obstacles, but instead of letting the obstacles crush them, they bust through them and come out stronger, all the while inspiring us. We don't always have the power to control what happens to us, or what challenges rise in our paths, but we do usually have a choice about how to react to the situation. Overcomers respond with grace and strength. They see complaining as a waste of time in a search for a solution. They will state the facts, but it is merely to describe the situation.

Overcomers see hope when they think a situation might be hopeless. They do not see giving up as an option. Their questions are about doing better and moving forward instead of asking why they are dealing with a challenge.

Overcomers teach us about strength and resilience. They show us there are things worth fighting for, and we should not settle for less than a joy-filled life.

Overcomers are fearless. They are the young entrepreneurs who follow their dreams, the athletes who keep pushing, those who don't accept the negative, and the ones who overcome the odds.

One of the stories I hear consistently at races is when someone uses running to prove he is going to overcome anything negative life throws his way. We were at a race that was raising money for breast cancer, and we had been talking to a woman in the registration line when a volunteer came over and gave her a new Keurig. I asked her why he had given her that and she told me everyone in the race who had cancer or who was a survivor was receiving a Keurig. I told her what an inspiration she was to be running while she was battling cancer, and she told me every time she could complete a run, it proved to her she could beat the disease, and that she was stronger than cancer. It was her way of fighting instead of feeling helpless.

At another race, I heard two amazing stories of overcomers. Maurice was a young man who had already had 15 operations to relieve pressure from fluid in his brain. He told me he runs to teach his daughters they should always have hope and never give up. He was not giving in to his medical issues. Roger came over to us and told us this was the first race he had run since his bowel surgery. He had to run with a colostomy bag, but he was excited because he could have that removed soon. I was amazed at these two inspirational people, and I kept thinking of all the people who find reasons not to exercise, but here was a man with a very good excuse to take some time off, but he refused to give in to a bump in the road.

Running can help you overcome grief. Sally told me the story of running helping her to overcome the grief of losing her mother. When I lost my oldest sister, I also lost my biggest supporter and my voice of reason. She always knew how I was feeling and exactly what words I needed to hear. I remember crying while running quite a few times while I overcame the grief from her death.

Running helped me overcome Covid. After my first round, I was still experiencing a lot of unusual fatigue even a month after Covid. I made a doctor's appointment, and he told me to push myself to the limit physically and make my lungs stronger, and not let this thing win. There have been many times since then when I want to stop running and I remember what he said, so I push through and run a mile or two more.

You cannot keep a runner down for long. While someone who faces a challenge might use it as an excuse to give up, a runner finds a way around the barrier. I remember a 5K where a man did the whole race with a walker. When you see that kind of determination it makes it hard to make excuses. At a race today, a woman asked me how old I was. When I told her I was sixty-four, she said she was forty-eight. She said, "Don't you find that you have more injuries as you age?" I said that had not been my experience, but I do have to take more preventive measures. Runners find a way.

I was watching the news today and they were talking about Asian hate crimes. They interviewed an Asian man who had decided to run a certain number of miles in order to "run through the hate" and to bring attention to the issue. We have so many stories like this. Remember the man who pushed his son in a stroller and ran because the son was disabled so he ran to give him the experience that his body would not allow? He found a way to overcome it.

I am including Raleigh in this chapter, too. After the first stroke, he drove his wife crazy by insisting that he had to walk nine miles each day while he was in the hospital because he didn't want to lose his fitness level. He would head off down the hall with his IV pole and his Garmin watch. He walked a six-mile race ten days after he left the hospital and I'm sure he would have run it except the woman doing the race with him was recovering from an injury and he didn't want to leave her alone. After the second stroke, the doctors discovered there was a hole in his heart that was probably causing the strokes. He had to have an operation, but it wasn't too long after that we were heading to a race. Raleigh lost partial sight in one eye after the first stroke, but instead of letting it bother him, he figured out how to work around it. There are running inspirations like Raleigh all around us.

Running can help overcome eating disorders. It can give you a focus on self-care, loving your body, and using food as fuel instead of control. It can offer a healthy sense of control.

Joshua's story

As runners, we often take running for granted. When an injury happens, we see what it is like to not be able to do our favorite activity, and sometimes our body let us know we need to find another form of exercise. However, imagine if running was never a choice for you because you physically could not perform it like others. Now imagine you are already being bullied and ridiculed because you don't fit into the box we describe as normal. Would you want to attempt something that would make the bullies pick on you worse? Joshua was not healed by running, but his story inspired many others to use it to tell his story and do what he could not.

Here is Joshua's story on a Facebook page on suicide prevention.

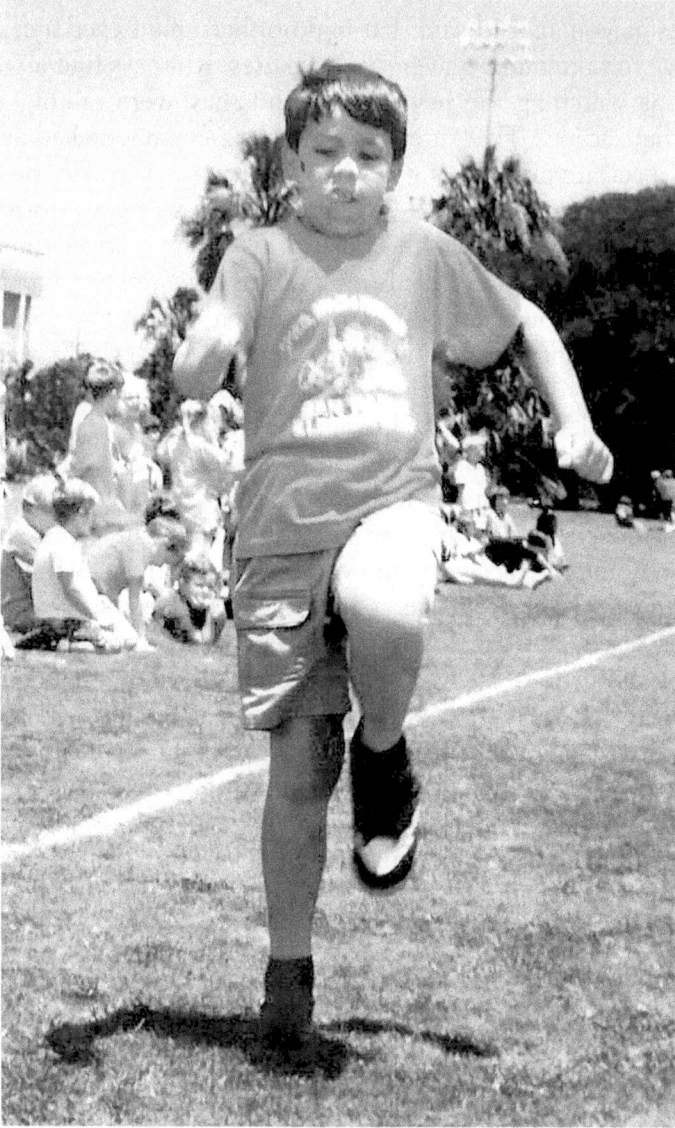

Joshua

Josh was the boy who wore corrective shoes as a child... walking wasn't always easy; running was even more difficult... something so many of us take for granted daily. He had put off taking a required physical education class until his junior year in high school, because he was so worried and intimidated by the requirements of the class. (A class most students take as a freshman, but mandatory for high school completion.)

Though we understand the significance of "requirements," we too often forget that not each of us is capable of the same things. We too often don't take the time to acknowledge that what is easy for some, is truly a burden for another. Too often, we don't realize what is happening in someone else's world.

Joshua's world was upside down. Nine months earlier he had lost his father, and time was running out on completing his mile for PE class, and he was a victim of bullying at school unbeknownst to his family. After having multiple conversations with his mom about having to run the mile and the seriousness of him not completing, it he was down to the wire, it had to be done that week. Joshua went off to school on a typical Tuesday. After arriving home from school that day, his mother, Ponda, asked him how it went. His reply was, "I ran that mile and it was the hardest thing I've ever done." His mom cooked him his favorite meal (cheeseburgers), and they sat together that evening and watched the Summer Olympics on television. On Wednesday morning when, Ponda went to wake him for school, she noticed Joshua's bed was made. Thinking he was already up and awake, moments later his mother realized he had never gone to bed. While she lay sleeping Joshua had taken his own life.

In the days that followed, Joshua's family went to his school to collect his belongings from his locker. That was when they learned of the bullying, and that day they learned that Joshua had never actually completed the mile that had worried, anguished and tortured him for years.

If you're capable of walking, running, or hiking a mile today, we ask that you do so for Joshua Waggoner and the many others just like him. Take the time today to reflect on how something we too often take for granted because *life* can change in an instant. Take the time to hug those closest to you a little longer, to tell those you haven't seen in a while that you care about them. Take the time to embrace doing something you might take for granted today, or not be able to do tomorrow. And most importantly, take the time to have a safe and meaningful conversation with those you love about suicide: share the message of Help, Hope and Life.

Feel free to post pictures of your walk/run/hike on Joshua's Mile 2015 FaceBook page http://tinyurl.com/josh2015run. So far today we've seen them coming in from the US, Egypt, Spain, and Afghanistan. There is also a t-shirt fundraiser that was designed for

Joshua's Mile 2015 for suicide prevention and awareness. All proceeds from the shirt sales are donated to the American Foundation for Suicide Prevention (Florida Chapter) in Joshua's memory. God Bless!

As today we celebrate the short life Joshua lived, don't forget to celebrate all the miles and memories you've been able to make. LIVE today.

If you or someone you know is in crisis, please call the Suicide Prevention Lifeline at 800-273-8255.

Here is the same story in his sister, Kim's, words:

> Running a mile is not difficult for me, but when I ran my mile for Joshua I realized that for others it may be the most difficult thing ever. Those words, One Mile, changed who I am. I'm sharing a moment in my life about a young man who had to wear corrective shoes within the first year of his life. As a teenager, he could walk but running was difficult. He tried but it was just awkward. The average person could not see his struggles because he looked normal, but the family knew it was hard on him.
>
> One of the courses required in high school to graduate is a year of P.E. Which means Josh would have to run.
>
> My brother, Joshua, put that off until his junior year because he was scared and stressed about it. A mile seemed to control him. He feared what others would say to him. He was teased in school because he was smart, gifted, and not a jock. He knew what running would or could do to him, but to graduate, he had to do it.
>
> One day during Junior year, he came home, and said to my mother, "Mom, I ran that mile today, it was the hardest thing I ever did."
>
> Little did she know that would be the last conversation they would have. Josh was only sixteen.
>
> As my family gathered his belongings at school, we were told he never made it to that gym class, he never ran that mile. Instead, he sat alone day in and day out and was teased by others because he was different.
>
> So yesterday, May 1st was his birthday, so I ran his mile for him.

Kim doesn't only run a mile for her brother, but also signs up for distance races that would challenge anyone, and then she crushes it one step at a time. Running the hard races helps her heal a little, and she knows how lucky she is to be capable of doing those races when others cannot.

My friend, Nancy, was going through her second battle with cancer when she asked me to do a race called Muddy Buddy with her. She wanted to prove cancer would not defeat her and that she could still compete. A Muddy Buddy race combines running and obstacles. Many of the obstacles are high and I have a fear of heights, but I would have done anything Nancy wanted at that point. You have to stay with your buddy for the whole race, and I didn't want to hold Nancy back. So, when I reached the top of each obstacle, I forced myself to go over to the other side without thinking. I remember when we reached one obstacle that required arm strength and Nancy was not able to do it. She looked at me and said, "Next year, I will be able to do that." I have always thought Nancy is one of the strongest women I know, and she showed her grit that day. I don't know too many people who can convince me to conquer my fear of heights, dive into a pool of mud, shimmy under barbed wire in mud, and climb up a rope to finish. The crazy thing is, I would do it again in a minute if she asked me.

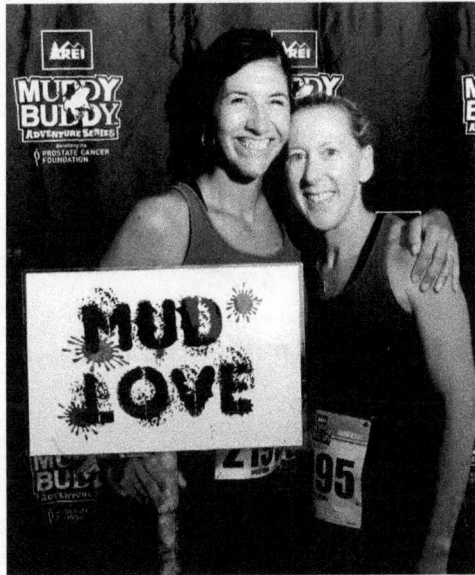

Nancy and I at The Muddy Buddy

Although I love music, I never listen to it during a race, because I want to hear the conversations around me. There are so many stories in every race. I often stand near the finish line and listen to what people say when they come across the line. Many are running to turn their health around, some are chasing a new goal, and others enjoy time with friends.

I see people who use running to overcome loneliness. Running can be a social activity, because there are local running clubs, and there are online running groups. When you come to a race, you will see what a social scene it is. Running can help you stay connected.

I have always thought laughter was a form of medicine, and my running adventures have proven this. We spend more time laughing before, during, and after running, and if you come to a race in a bad mood, you will not leave the same way.

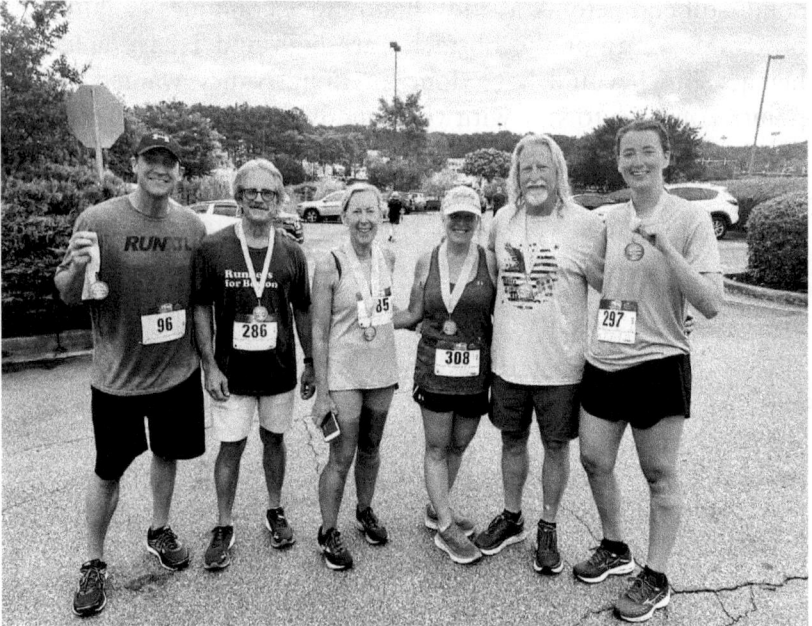

Some of the good friends I have made because of the running community.

4   Running for Physical Healing

Most people would agree that runners are generally in good physical condition. I always think more people should come to races and be inspired by the variety of people who use running to become stronger. I also wish more people knew what it can do for you physically, and how those benefits translate into making your life better. Here are a few of the benefits:

It helps to build strong bones, because it is a weight-bearing exercise.

- It improves cardiovascular fitness.
- Improves your memory.
- Gives you better mood and energy.
- Maintains a healthy weight.
- Improves sleep.
- Improved knee and back health.
- Increased lung capacity.
- It improves your immunity.
- It improves mental health.

Running for at least ten minutes a day can lower your risk of cardiovascular disease. It lowers your resting heart rate. The lower the rate, the more efficient your heartbeat. It helps you to sleep better and your body repairs itself when you are asleep.

Running for thirty minutes can trigger your immune system to help you feel better. It boosts your mood, concentration, and energy. It improves your knee and back health. It improves your memory.

Running provides cognitive benefits including working memory, focus, and task switching.

Paula tells us how running helped improve her health: "My first race was a wake-up call that I needed to get in shape. I told myself that I never wanted to feel like that again, tired, fat, sore, and ashamed that those three miles were so hard." Running can improve you physically and add years to your life.

My proof of what running does for me physically happens anytime I go to the doctor. One of the visits I will never forget happened when I had to go to urgent care after Karate class when I had popped my stitches from a skin cancer surgery. The nurse asked me for a list of medications I was taking. I told him I wasn't using anything. He asked me two more times if I was sure. This tells me that he is used to hearing a long list from most people. I know running has kept me from needing medication.

I also pay attention to the physical state of other people my age and older, and I don't have to be a doctor to tell you that if you do not move your body, you will lose your mobility. This means you will not be able to move around independently and enjoy a good quality of life. There is truth in "move it or lose it." I have seen runners in their eighties who run in races and look like they are enjoying every minute.

Running has helped me learn more about my body, its limits, and what it needs to function well. I started to run ultras and I was fascinated by how my body reacted to long distances. I made every mistake in the book, but I asked lots of questions from experts and I tried to learn from each mistake. Running allows you to challenge yourself.

Running can give you the confidence you need in tough situations. Over time, you will strengthen your body and see performance improvements. It makes the impossible seem more possible. Confidence will carry over to other areas of your life.

Running teaches you resilience. There will be setbacks in your running career, but you will learn how to rise back up and try something different. Most runners have had at least one injury, but they don't give up because of this roadblock. They do what they can, and when they heal, they start running again.

Running proves to you how you can improve your abilities with practice and hard work. The improvements you can see from running are tangible evidence. One day, you can barely run a mile, but in a month, you are running three and planning on doing more mileage. I remember a runner at a half-marathon who said,

"Running is a gateway drug, one minute you are doing a 5k, and then you are doing 150 miles across a desert."

Hal describes how running saved him physically. "My wife was pregnant in the summer of 1995. She gained weight, but so did I. I got up to 212 lbs., on a 5'9" frame. I was smoking cigarettes, drinking soda, eating out...anything that destroys your body.

In the spring of 1997, I was walking around a home goods store with my family, and I started experiencing chest pains. We drove to the hospital, and it was explained to me that I had suffered a small cardiac "event." It absolutely scared me to no end! A couple of weeks later my grandfather passed away from emphysema. On top of my recent "event," I had to make some SERIOUS changes! I was always an athlete growing up. I played baseball, basketball, and football. I always enjoyed running. So I decided to stop eating out and put cigarettes down.

Honestly, though, it was about to get easy. I went on a deployment in the Navy that summer. The first night out to sea, I thought I would get on a treadmill. I was running at a decent pace but couldn't finish an entire mile without being completely worn out and breathless. I continued extending my distance each night, while choosing to eat fruit and cutting out soda and fatty foods. By the end of the 6-month deployment, I was running over 8 miles a night. I lost 30 lbs. When I got back, I didn't stop running. I decided to sign up for races in central California. I would run one a month. Then I moved to San Diego in 2000 and started running races more frequently. I was running three or four races a month. I've continued running since then. I've taken time off here and there from running races, but still run nearly every day. Last year, I ran fifty races. I never picked up smoking again, I don't drink soda, and I've been fortunate enough to get my heart rate to a level that my cardiologist called a Runner's Heart. Running gives me energy, keeps my spirits high, introduces me to great friends, and keeps the weight off.

The running community is without a doubt the most supportive community there is. I have met so many amazing people along the way!

I'm thankful that I can continue on because I know the day will come where I have to slow up, or even worse, stop."

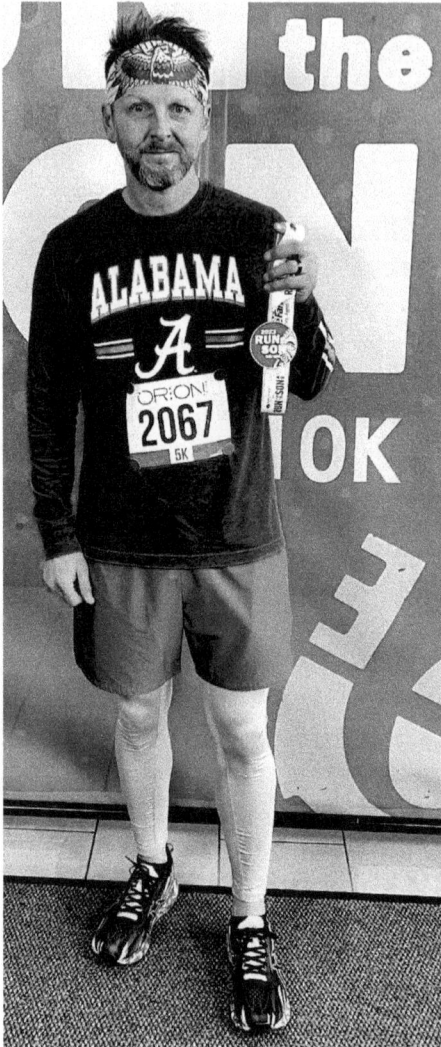
Hal with one of his many medals

I met Norman at a race today where the race director told his story. Here is his journey in his own words:

"I've always been a physical guy, working construction in my early years, and keeping a hand in it when I began designing houses. Forty was fast approaching when I was diagnosed with multiple sclerosis (MS), which can be severely crippling. Eight years passed with the disease progressing and no clear solutions. Then my daughter asked me to begin walking with her to help with her lacrosse training and fitness. While she was away at camp, I got bored walking alone and started jogging a bit. Before I knew it, I was running three miles at a time! Then my daughter talked me into entering a 5k at her middle school. I was stunned when I won second in my age group! Soon my college-age daughter encouraged me to enter a race in her college town. Second in my age group again and I received my award from NFL running back and Georgia Southern alum) Adrian Peterson!! I'd found something I enjoyed that I was good at, and I was hooked.

I have recently celebrated three-and-a-half years since my first race. I've just passed the 468th race, including 5k, 10k, several half-marathons, and even two marathons. I've moved on to a different age group now, but I still enjoy bringing home those medals—even a couple of grandmasters!

While exercise can't cure MS, keeping my mind and body in top condition helps to reduce the long-term effects of a relapse, and thankfully, with recent advances in medical research, I'll be able to get out there with my running mates for many more years."

Running helps you to learn how to tap into willpower and self-control. You can learn how to push through pain and fatigue. I remember a half-marathon I did several years ago. It was a trail race, and the terrain was a little crazy. There was one corner with a thirty-foot drop-off, so you didn't want to take that turn too hard. There were other spots where there was a short, extreme incline that you had to

Norman at a local race

shimmy and crawl over. It was slightly brutal, but I didn't fall until there were only five miles to go. I had been talking and not paying attention, and my foot hooked on a root, and I was going downhill, so not only did I fall, I slid. It didn't hurt, but I had blood all over my arm and leg. When we approached the last aid station, the volunteers both looked horrified and asked if I wanted a medic. I just smiled and said, "Oh, no. It happens all the time." You learn to keep going and bring a first-aid kit.

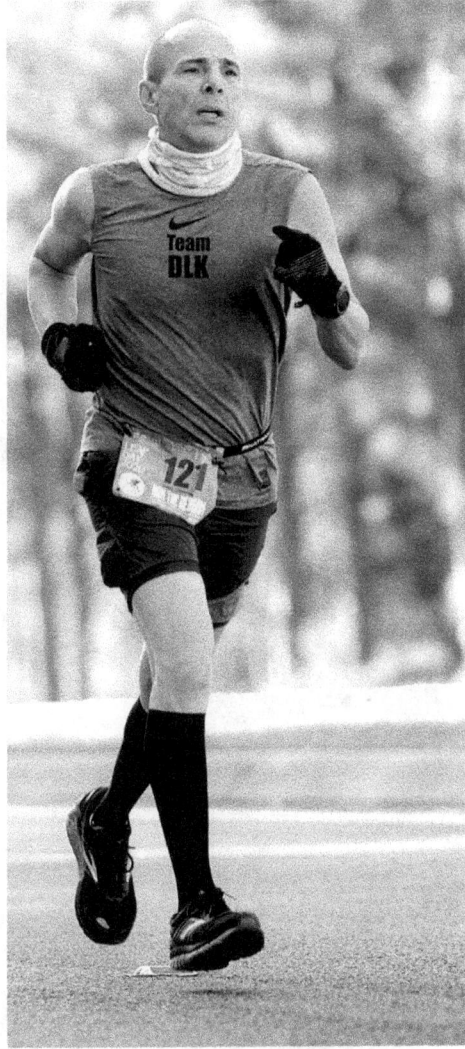

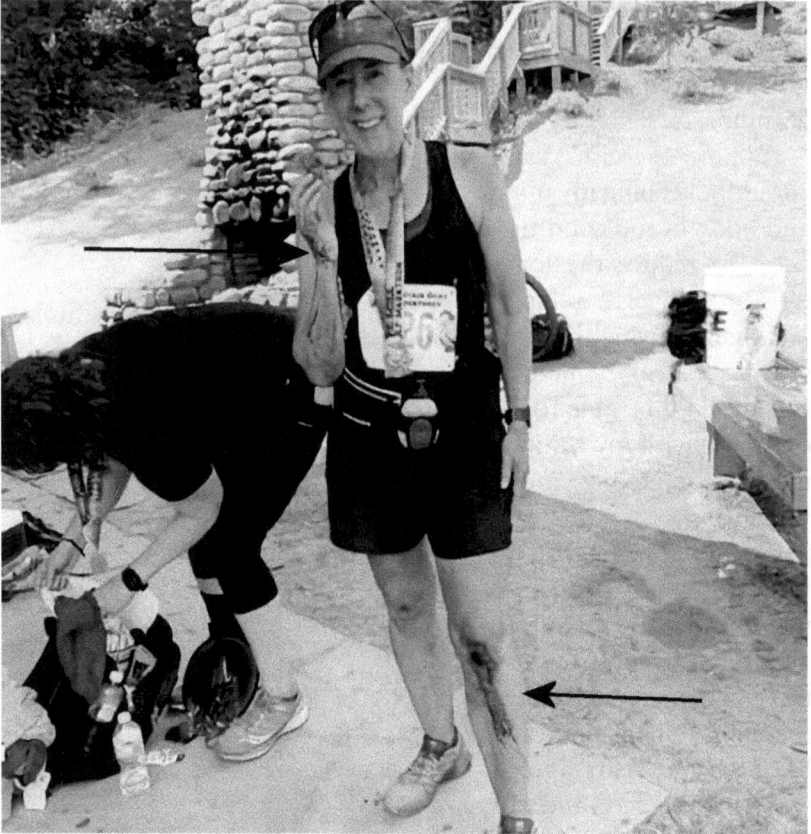

Another race where I fell on the trail!

Running can teach you to appreciate challenging experiences. This happened when I was running downhill, and I was talking to the two people I had been running with for most of the race. I wasn't paying attention, and my foot got caught on a root, so not only did I fall, I slid several feet. I had a huge cut, and when I crossed the finish line the medic looked at it and said, "Oh my, you need to get this looked at." It was fine.

Listen to this story by a writer on Medium called "Banned Filename Jr." about his use of running to heal both physically and mentally.

"Some of my strongest childhood memories involve running. This may not surprise those who know me as a guy who runs five kilometers each day, competes in marathons, and is hoping to leap into the ultra-running world this year. But if you knew me as a child beset by severe asthma, you may be wondering how I got here.

"From a very young age I was considered fragile, an unathletic child due to my health issues — and in this instance, I tapped into a special sort of determination, one borne of an early tetchiness over the stigma of being a non-athlete. Though my mother was nervous, I was single-mindedly determined to defy the limits of my health condition.

"But then I dropped the thread. Several asthma attacks requiring hospitalization all but killed any prospects I may have had as a track and field standout, and it would be nearly two decades until I'd run for the joy of it. I all but accepted my destiny as a non-athlete and spent the next few decades living almost exclusively inside my brain, focusing on artistic and academic pursuits. My legs were relegated to a form of transportation that got me from class to class, from band practice to drama classes to friends' houses to get high and watch movies.

"My non-athletic self-image was further compounded by a car accident at age 17. I was left with a bad ankle fracture. While rehab was relatively straightforward, and the recovery time probably contributed to my excellent marks in Grade 12 (I wasn't getting out much), it all but galvanized my new self-image: all-brain, no body. I was an egghead, and there was nothing to do but push forward with intellectual pursuits.

"At the worst of my 2014 depression and anxiety attacks, running seemed to be the only thing that would break the cloud cover. Marathons could not have been further from my mind. My objective was survival, from one day to the next. Doing what I needed to ensure basic human functionality.

"It wasn't until 2016 that I truly began to realize the healing power of running very long distances. I'd quit drinking, was struggling to stay sober and had recently lost my job — and these forces seemed intent on dragging me back into the abyss of depression. I began to focus on my running. Gradually, and without really intending to, I increased my distances. And then, on a random sunny spring weekday, I went for my usual run and just kept going. It was only after I'd gotten home that, out of curiosity, I calculated my distance on Google Maps. I'd just run a half-marathon.

"I *do* think there's an argument to be made for combating mental illness with some form of physical exertion. The head is inseparable from the rest of the human body, and what's good for the body is invariably good for the head.

"In my experience, no medication even comes close to strenuous physical exercise when it comes to fostering psychological equanimity. If I were to stop taking my antidepressants tomorrow and keep running, I have no doubt there would be challenges, but I'm reasonably confident I would be fine. But keep me from running for more than two days and I'm a considerably crankier person, even with the benefit of drugs. The most powerful medicine lives within me."

5   Running for Mental Healing

When I began this book, I sent out a request for stories from anyone who had something to say about how running had affected him or her. Most of the stories involved mental healing. I find it interesting that a sport we think of as a physical activity has affected so many people more mentally than physically.

Running can help with anxiety and depression. It is proven that running is as effective as antidepressant medication. My friend, Kim, was struggling with severe depression and was seeing a doctor

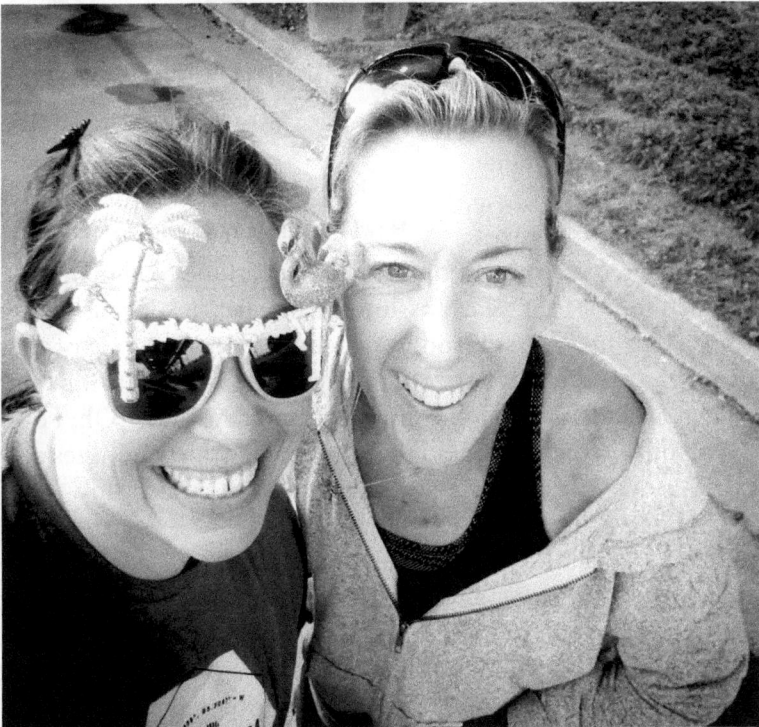

Kim and I at a local race.

every week. She felt very alone, but as she started to run, the negative thoughts lifted. Running can give someone hope, and the running community is very loving and supportive. The friends she made through running made her feel valued and loved. Kim says that running saved her life. I was surprised when Kim told me this because when I met her, she was full of joy and energy. She seemed happy and she loved running. Kim calls herself *Kim Possible* like the cartoon character who takes on all kinds of danger and crushes it. Because of running, Kim now crushes negativity. I am so thankful to know her.

Another friend, Howie, uses running as stress

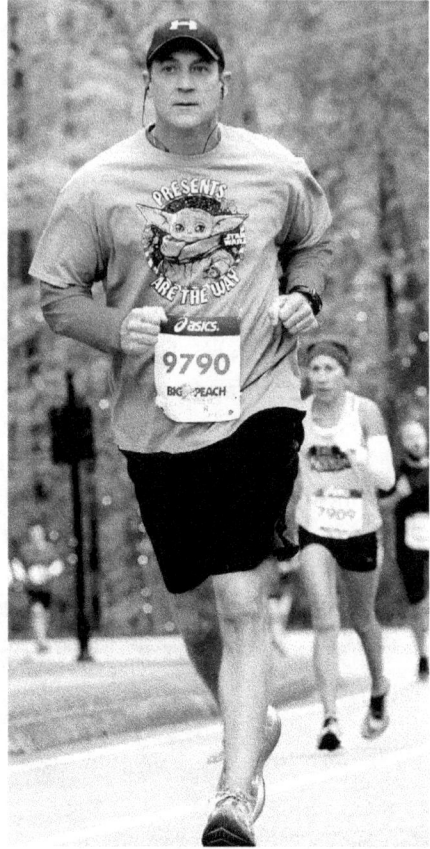

Howie on his way to another medal

relief. He says, "What started simply as something to help me relax has turned into a four-year passion for me. It has kept me healthy and has given me a great group of friends." Howie is one of those runners who is naturally fast. I wanted to learn his secrets for speed, but when I asked him what he did for training he said, "Oh, I don't run at all during the week. I do the elliptical for thirty minutes a few days a week. I was running every day, but was so much slower than him, so that was not what I wanted to hear!

When I was taking karate, I met a man named Joe who was an editor for the local paper and wrote several books about the history of Marietta, Ga. Joe was an athlete, but that was an identity that did not come easily to him. His body kept giving him challenge after challenge. He ran races and did karate with only one lung. He

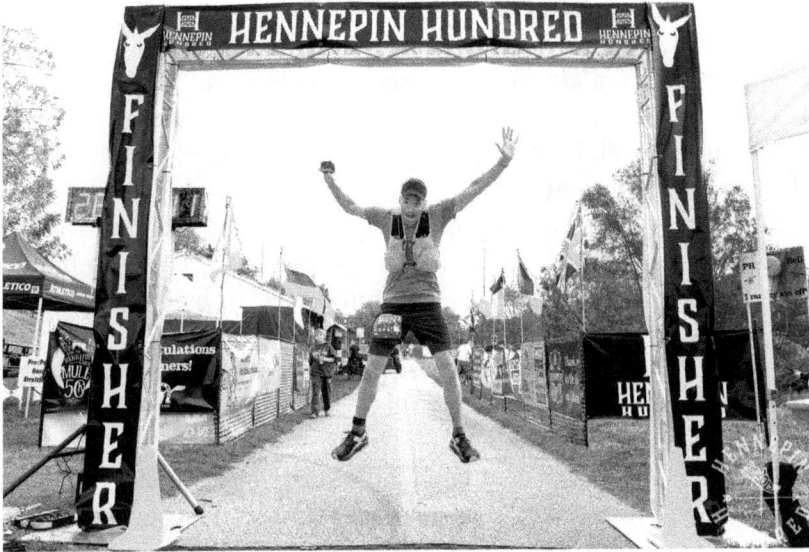

Trey as he completes another amazing feat.

refused to make excuses or give up. He just kept rising and doing his best. He was an inspiration to us all and we loved his sense of humor. Joe died from cancer, but I guarantee you that it wasn't without a fight. His sister, Susan, told me she runs because of him. This is what she said, "I run because it lets me be with my brother who ran. It was something he enjoyed that saved his life in many ways. When I run I think about him."

Trey is one of those runners who many people classify as crazy. He repeatedly runs 100-mile races and comes up with ideas like "Let's run 75 miles of the Appalachian Trail for fun." He is also one of the sweetest men I know and his love for running is contagious. Here is what he says about running: "Running gives me a connection with nature. It helps me clear my mind. Whatever I was upset about at mile one will seem less heavy by mile six. Running is spiritual for me. Some of my best conversations with God have been on long runs. I have to be worn down to let go and listen to God."

I agree with Trey about the conversations with God. I run in my neighborhood, and I talk out loud to God, even though it's more muttering, but I always wonder if my neighbors think I'm crazy because I'm talking to the air. I also work out problems when I'm running. There is something about movement that helps me to think better. Here is an article I wrote about running with God.

Running is the time during the day when I find a sense of peace and calm. Even during races, there is a time when everything seems silent and peaceful as everyone becomes spaced out along the road.

During this peaceful time, I have my best conversations with God. I usually tell Him how much I need His help in all things, and if He can just be patient with me, I will try to follow where He leads. I also ask Him to make any messages He has for me abundantly clear because sometimes I need neon lights to understand what I should do. I end my conversations by asking God to use me as He needs me. I occasionally add "If you can, just give me some warning!" I have been blindsided many times by people who had unexpected serious needs, and I had to think fast to try to help them.

Running also helps me to do God's work. I love interacting with people, and I think strangers can sense this openness because I seem to attract people who need to tell their stories. I love that people do this because I love hearing stories, and most people need someone who will listen. They need to share their burdens and telling someone else lessens those burdens a little. When I feel like I am helping people, I know I am doing God's work. At races, there are so many stories to be told of people struggling in one way or another. Some are trying to lose weight, some are running to prove they are stronger than an illness, and some are just looking for social interaction.

God uses running to show me inspiration as well. When I see someone with a huge leg brace ambling along, or someone with another challenge who shows up without excuses, it makes me want to try harder.

I believe God is with me on my runs in the peacefulness I feel as I cruise along or the personal interactions I have with other runners. I cannot imagine a better running partner.

I use running as an escape. I use it to run away from a bad day, judgment, toxic people, a tough situation, a decision I can't make, sadness, or frustration.

I also have runs when I clear my mind of everything, and only take in what's around me. I let my mind have a rest. I spoke with a man this weekend who agrees with me. We had just finished a 5K, so we still had our race bibs on, and we were walking around an arts festival. We stopped at a booth where the woman said her husband used to run. I started talking with him and discovered he had stopped because he had injured his foot badly while trail running. I asked him if he missed it, and he said, "Oh, absolutely. I loved heading out on the trail and focusing on the path in front of me. It was a chance to forget everything else. I could let my mind go blank and enjoy the nature around me."

Michael is a veteran runner and an ambassador for a local race organization. He sums up how running affects us:

"We all run for different reasons and have different goals. Even an individual's running purpose is likely to change throughout their running life. Through the years, I've run for speed, I've run for consistency, I've run for Fellowship, I've run for love, I have run to clear my mind, I've run to communicate with my higher power, and I've run to have some sort of control in my life at times when everything seemed out of kilter. I have run to beat others, and I have run to beat myself. These are

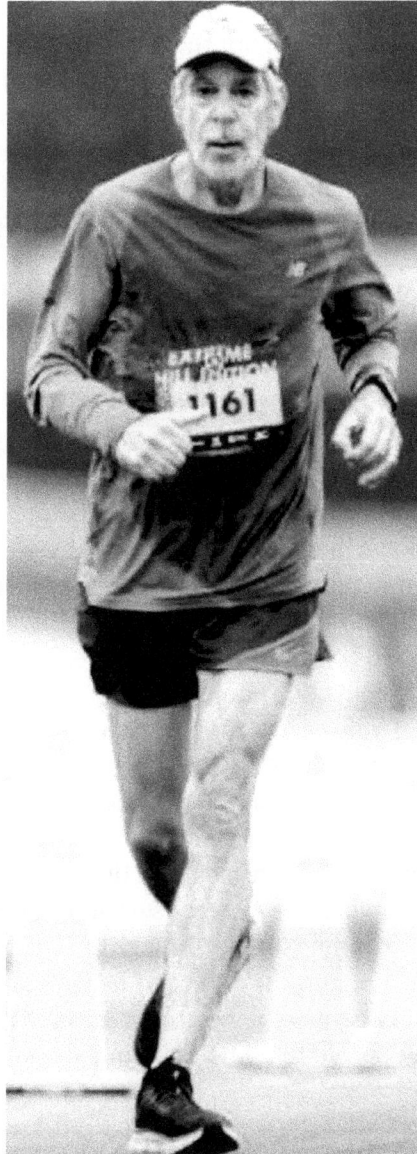

Michael enjoying a race

only some of the reasons I have run. There are others as well.

I have been running for over forty years, and honestly, I think that sometimes I run simply because I have forgotten how to not run. it is so ingrained in me that when I don't do it for periods of time, I get restless and feel the need for the kind of movement that only a run can satisfy.

I am not the runner I used to be, but I wouldn't expect anything different. I am not the person I used to be either, but hopefully, the person I am becoming is better than the person I was. I can say the same about running. Even though I will never run faster than I have in the past, and I will never run longer than I have in the past, it does not mean my running won't improve, and it will, as long as its purpose shines more brightly as time goes on. at my age, every run is a privilege. There have been younger days when I couldn't run, which makes the ability to do so even more valued today than ever before.

I'm racing tomorrow morning, but I won't be racing. More accurately, I'll be attending an event surrounded by a bunch of good friends I already know, and potential friends I still have to meet. For me, right now, that is the most important thing."

I know one of the reasons running is mentally healing, because it allows me to be out in nature. My neighbors think I'm crazy when I'm out running in the drizzle, but I love running in the rain, and taking in the quiet around me. Being outside and listening to all the sounds of nature is peaceful to me. I can feel stress melt away when I am outside running.

I am also the most creative when I am running. My mind is clear, and no one is asking me questions. I can work out problems and come up with several different ideas for articles.

It can build mental toughness. You see what you can do, and it builds your confidence. You see that you are the type of person who can overcome obstacles. You learn to trust yourself.

Running breaks down barriers. Runners are quick to share their stories, and they want to hear yours.

Laughter can be great medicine to help with your mental health. Let me share a few moments of our laughter on the road.

- Sally and I were running a race at a church where the pastor came out to bless the runners. He was wearing his vestment, and Sally told him she liked his scarf.

- At my first ultra, I asked a man what his name was. He said, "Cornbread." At that moment I decided I needed an ultra-name. I still haven't decided what it should be.

- My husband wanted to help me with the ultras, but when he arrived with two coffees and a sandwich, he fell on the hill, both coffees flew in the air, and he landed on the sandwich. I felt bad for him, and I was sad about the coffees, but I couldn't stop laughing.

- I was running a race that was called just an ultra (26.6 miles) and I had a migraine and a bad attitude from the start. I knew I was close to finishing, so I decided to check at the table to see how many more laps I had, then I would go to the bathroom and finish my laps. They told me I had five laps to go, and the woman in the lead was half a lap ahead of me. I started sprinting, passed the woman, and said, "Good job!" and only stopped to catch my breath now and then until the end. That was a glorious win.

There are so many more times filled with laughter. The laughter begins moments after my running friends are together. The laughter lifts my spirits as much as running does.

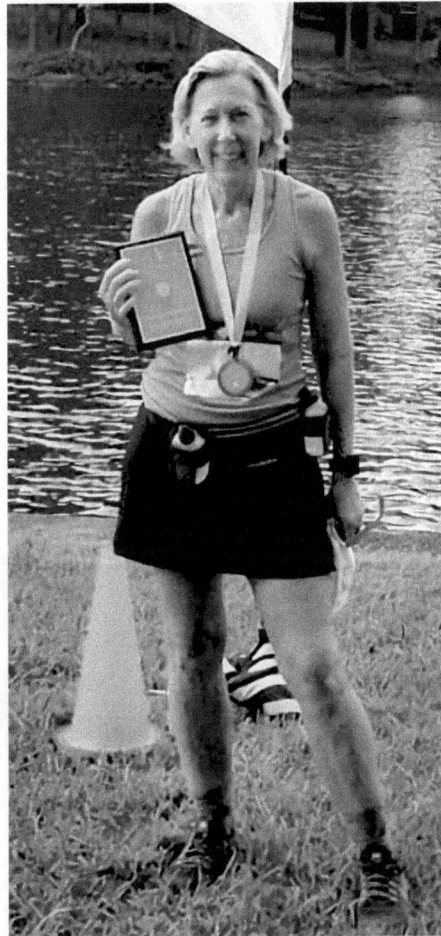

My first win at an ultra-marathon

6   Running for Social Healing

If you are feeling lonely for any reason, you should start signing up for local races or join a local running club. It doesn't matter if you need to move like a snail, the goal is to become a part of the running community, which will provide you with new friendships and connections. It will also inspire you to push yourself, because runners are inspirational. They are some of the nicest people you can meet, and I am always happy to see how friendly and open they are. When you go to a race, the chances are good you are going to make at least one connection, and you will hear many stories. Runners like to support and encourage, and who doesn't need more of that in his life? Everyone is welcome in the running community, and other runners want to hear your running story and share theirs as well.

Going to a race often feels like attending a family event. Strangers wander over to each other and start conversations, runners exchange their reasons for running, and share their running experiences.

I met my best friends because of running. Sally came up to me during a kickboxing class at the gym. She told me she saw me running on the track all the time and she wanted to start running, so she asked me to start doing races with her. I met Robbin at the gym and thought she was the nicest woman I had ever met. I met Raleigh at a race he had come to with Robbin, and I met Kim because of her friendship with Robbin. They are good friends I can rely on to be there. There are many others I can add to the list, because runners are good people.

Sally told me she wanted to meet people. I told her that going to races was the fastest way to do that. I was surprised that Sally was having trouble meeting people because she is funny and full of energy, but she wasn't confident about speaking to people at first. I guarantee you that many years later, this is not the case anymore!

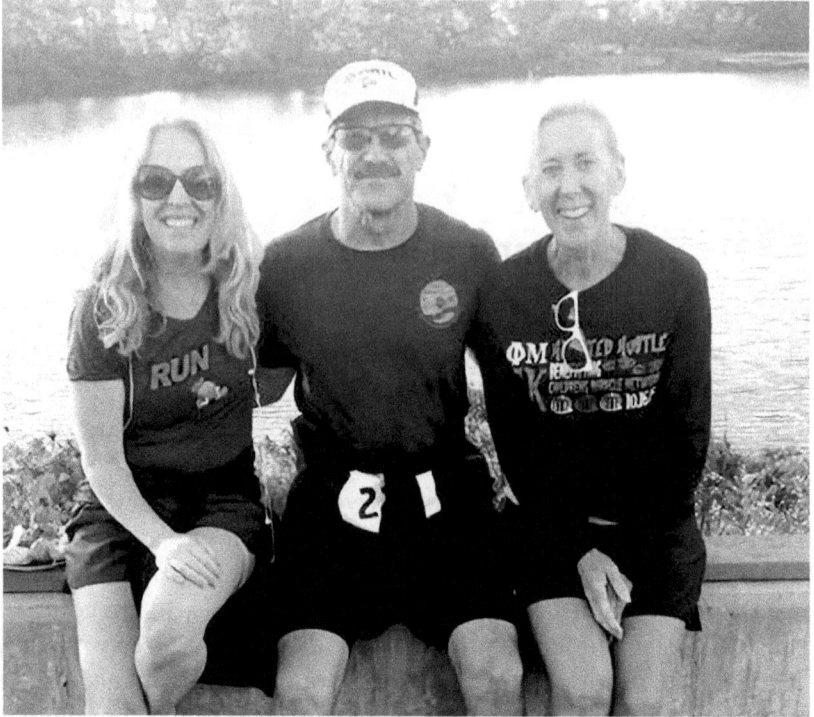

Sally, Raleigh, and I at a Halloween race

Once as we were standing around after a race, a handsome man approached us and said to Sally, "Are you Kate?" The once shy Sally answered, "I could be." Everyone on the race circuit knows Sally, and if you don't, you are missing out.

There have been so many healing moments with these four people. I have laughed until my stomach hurt and shared my most vulnerable moments. Having people like this in your life is healing because you know you have their support no matter what happens.

When I was coaching, there was a social element to each practice. As we waited for everyone to show up, I listened to what the runners did that day. There were plenty of stories and lots of laughter. There was a blueberry orchard near where we ran and at the end of some practices, we feasted on blueberries while we planned our strategy for the next race.

What I loved the most though was how many runners stayed after practice to run easy loops on our running trail while we talked about everything on our minds. Those runs were healing for them too.

Our friend, Kim, was going through some tough times, and she needed to feel that she had the support of friends. At one race, Raleigh and I went back on the course to run in with her, and this picture reminds us of our bond.

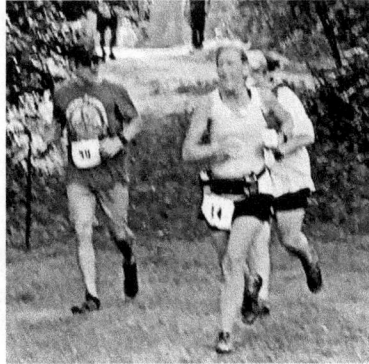

Running clubs give members a chance to form important communities. One of these groups is called "Paulding Sole Mates." It is a group of women who train to run together. Anyone is welcome to join, regardless of fitness level. They encourage each other and often come as a whole group to races. When you run with a group, it can motivate you to run consistently because you feel more accountable about showing up. When you are encouraging someone else it makes you feel as if you are supporting other runners. Having a running family is healing.

At almost every race, I come away with a new connection. I was at a trail half-marathon, and I was nervous because the race organizer was known to run very tough races. I started running and found myself behind a group of women who were going to do the whole run together. One person had country music playing quietly while they talked about all kinds of things. There was laughter and encouragement, and the pace they were going was perfect for me. I asked them if they would adopt me, and I became known as our new friend Jen. I ran with them for quite a while until they stopped for a photo opportunity. I wanted to continue, so I thanked them and said I was going to keep going. One of the women said she would like to go with me, so we headed off down the trail. Sarah was twenty-four and this was her first half-marathon. I commented that she picked a tough course for her first one, but I think we helped each other through the run. There were a few spots where we laughed because the terrain was so rugged, but we shared each other's stories. I finished that day feeling inspired by a young woman who was not afraid to do something hard. I believe God puts people in your life at the exact moment you need them, or they need you. What better place to meet them than out on a quiet trail in the woods?

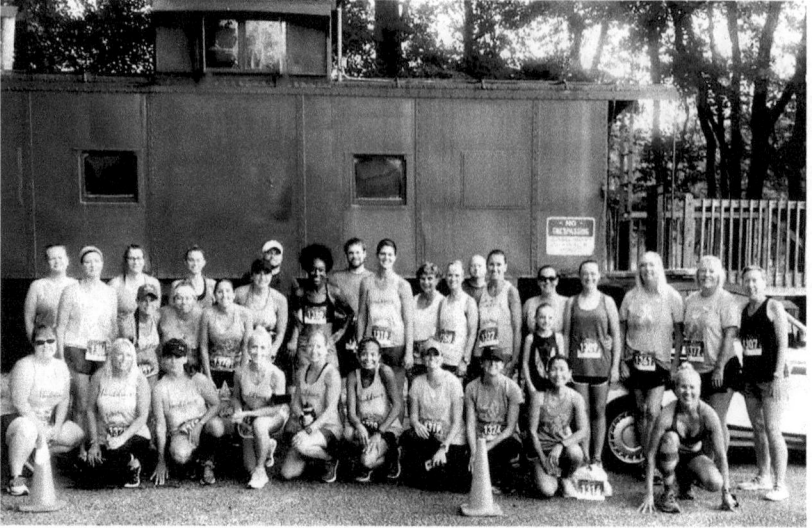

The Paulding Sole Mates.

Here is a quote from Jeff Galloway describing the social impact of running. "I had gotten to know some of the other lazy kids, and they said that winter cross-country was the one to do because you could lie to the coach and tell him you were going to run on the trails, and you could go out to the edge of the woods and hide out. I did that for two days and then an older kid I liked came up to me and said, "Galloway, you're running with us today." I guess I'd been busted. I ran with them, and I was going to drop out at the woods, but they were funny, and they told interesting stories and gossiped about the teachers as they ran. I stayed as long as I could, but I couldn't run very far that first day. I got hooked during those ten weeks on the social aspect of running and the way I felt empowered."

One of the other aspects I love about the social side of running is how friendly competition with friends can make you a better runner. Sally, Raleigh, and I are good friends, but we are always doing our best to beat each other, and that positive competition pushes us to be better. Our competitive spirit has also provided us with laughter and funny stories.

Raleigh and I were doing a half-marathon and I stopped at the bathroom at least three times, so Raleigh was sure he would win. I slowly decreased the distance between us until he was right in front of me. I could tell he was struggling by the way he was running, and he was giving himself a pep talk. When Raleigh is not running well he starts talking to himself to get motivated. I pulled up next to him and said in the cheeriest, not out of breath at all voice, "Hi buddy!" I will never forget the look on his face. It was part disbelief and part defiance. He looked at me and said, "Oh, hell no!" and he took off. I couldn't chase him because I was laughing so hard. There were a few runners who were looking at us and wondering what just happened.

At another race, Raleigh was injured and was not going to run, but as I was checking in I saw him looking at the registration table, and I knew he wanted to participate. I told him if he wanted to do the race, I would stay with him. We could run slowly or walk. We were going at a slow, steady pace when we saw Sally ahead of us. I looked at Raleigh and said, "I don't want you to hurt yourself, but can you run fast enough so we can pass her?" He replied, "Oh, there is no way I would miss this opportunity." As we passed we both said, "Hi, Sally." I can't repeat what she said to us.

Once, I thought Sally could use some company, so I said, "Sally, do you want to run together?" She said she did, so we ran the whole race together, and as we came close to the finish line I said to Sally, "Let's finish together." Her response was to sprint across the line ahead of me yelling, "I beat Jen!" All is fair in a competition.

There is often trash-talking between us at the races, and often even as we train. Raleigh always wants to beat me in how many steps he has, so I often text him and tell him how many I have and that I hope he isn't sitting on the sofa eating bonbons. I always hope I am motivating him to keep pushing to improve, and he does the same for me.

Running can also help you bond with family. My friend, Rachel, is training for a marathon with her dad. She wrote on Facebook that it doesn't matter who finishes first. The time spent with her dad as they train together is priceless. Imagine all the conversations and laughter they will have as they log the miles. Here is what she said, "My daddy and I have been running races together for years. We have similar paces and are both incredibly competitive, so we motivate each other to do our best or die trying. He wins some races, and I win others. Our after-race photos often have us mocking the other with the winner proudly holding up a #1. We have raced multiple half marathons together, but never full. I have only run one full marathon, and it was fourteen years ago. My dad has never run one. This is a milestone year for both of us; I turn forty in March, and he turns seventy in April. I know he has always wanted to do a marathon, and I've wanted to do another one. I called him at the new year and told him we were doing it this year. I knew our competitive drives would have us ready if we knew we were both doing it, and so far my plan is working. Dad ran 15.1 miles Monday, and he had never run further than 13.1. I love that my dad and I share our love for running (and for beating each other, lol); it brings us closer and makes us better."

Running has so many benefits beyond what it can do for us physically. We all can do better with a community to support us, and the running community is one of the best.

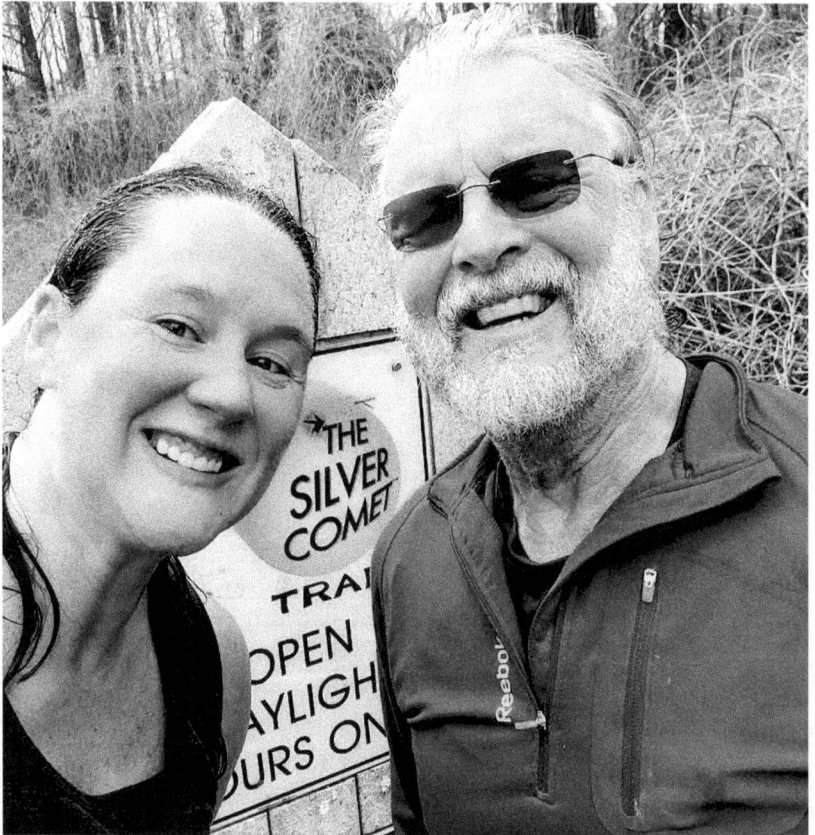

Rachel and her dad.

7   Running to Heal Self-Image

I am very critical of myself, and I often feel like I am not very good at most things. Running was different. When I was younger, I was fast, and I have always had endurance for longer races. It was something I was good at doing. When I'm running, I feel strong and powerful. It makes me feel free.

Our mental and physical health are connected and have to be in balance for us to be our best. Running can help us with anger, stress, anxiety and depression, and once we are healing our mind, we can begin to see the beauty in our body. Exercise can help us see our possibilities. We suddenly realize we are capable of much more than we thought. We can set goals, bust through them, and make new ones. We have tangible evidence that we are improving.

Running gives us a connection to our bodies. You start to focus more on being strong and healthy than worrying about your weight. Instead of being so focused on how you look, you begin to think more about how you feel. My friend, Sally, used to restrict her calories because she did not want to gain weight. We all know if you restrict those calories too much it can be dangerous. When Sally started running, she began to see herself as the athlete she is, and her relationship with food became much healthier.

Leigh Weingus' article, "7 Reasons Running Improves Confidence," states there is a link between goal setting and confidence.

When you start to identify yourself as a runner, you also identify with the qualities of a runner which are grit, resilience, and persistence.

Running shows us anything is possible with patience and hard work.

There is a running organization called "261 Fearless." Their goal is to empower women by giving them the confidence to do epic things. The name comes from Katherine Switzer's bib number. She was the first woman to run the Boston marathon in 1967, and a race official tried to pull her off the course. She faced her fear and completed her goal. A team of men and women are working on projects that enable women to take personal responsibility for healthy and sustainable change within their lives. It offers women's education and women's running opportunities to discover their self-worth and potential and discover ways to make choices to control their lives.

Another organization is "Back on My Feet," which helps people who are homeless and struggling with addiction to build confidence, accountability, and other life skills through running. Participants make a commitment to run three times a week. The non-profit gives participants new running shoes after their third consecutive run. The national program began in 2007 in Philadelphia, and now has chapters in seventeen cities. It partners with shelters and centers for addiction and recovery for the homeless. The goal of the program is to create a community and opportunity for members to have a positive influence in their lives, and a way to build their confidence.

One member commented that he needed an outlet to clear his mind and have something to focus on instead of the negatives in his life. This running club offers members a chance to talk with others who are going through similar struggles. They can talk with mentors and receive help and education. One member, Montavious, said, "I had been living that street life. Drugs, gangs. I wanted to change. It helped me develop meaningful relationships and connections. I learned to trust people again. There are people out there who love me and just want to see you win."

"Still I Run" is a running community that promotes running to benefit mental health while working to erase the stigma, raise awareness about the topic, and help others run for mental health. This is a quote from their web page:

"Because one of the best ways to help combat anxiety and depression (aside from medication and therapy) is through exercise and running. We combine the two. The name 'Still I Run' is inspired by the famous Maya Angelou poem, *Still I Rise*. Though we may feel defeated and deflated, we can fight the good fight and get out and be healthy, both physically and mentally... together."

Organizations like these understand the healing power of running. They know running can change the image you have of yourself. It proves to you that you can improve with hard work and commitment, and it gives you confidence. It gives you a sense of success, which some people have never experienced before.

To build a strong self-image with running, don't compare yourself to other runners. Run your own race and set your own goals. Anyone who is competitive wants to improve her performance, but sometimes you have to be happy with doing your best. I have some very fast friends and sometimes it can be frustrating to know I cannot do what they do. Let me introduce you to a few. Anna is not only super-fast, but she also gets up at 4 a.m. to run distance. Every day her social media post details her run, and I use them to motivate me because if Anna can run sixteen miles at 4 a.m., I can manage three later in the day. Hal is an elite runner who usually finishes in the top five. He is also very humble for someone with that much running talent.

I do not compare myself to these friends, and I cheer them on, because running has something to offer everyone no matter when you cross the finish line.

When runners are asked how running heals self-image, they reply by saying that running has made them respect their bodies and what they are capable of doing. It also proves that if you can run, you are made of tough stuff. When you have increasing feelings of accomplishment, you feel less critical of yourself.

Running can start a domino effect where you start doing positive things for your body, you start feeling better, and you begin to see your body differently.

When you run, you have feelings of accomplishment, which translates into feeling better about yourself.

Endorphins trigger a positive feeling that can lead to a positive outlook on life.

Others encouraging you and commenting on your achievements can raise your self-esteem.

Professor Kathleen Martin Ginis comments on a body image study she did, "We think that the feelings of strength and empowerment women achieve post exercise stimulate an improved internal dialogue. This, in turn, should generate positive thoughts and feelings about their bodies which may replace the all-too-common negative ones."

Set goals for your running, celebrate your accomplishments, reflect on your hard work, and be proud of yourself. Having an exercise plan and sticking to it is an accomplishment in itself.

8   Healing Through Inspiration

One of the reasons I love to go to races is I always walk away inspired, and I am as inspired by the people in the back as I am by the ones in the front.

I always admire the amount of work the elite runners put into their training and how willing they are to share their wisdom with other runners. Their fitness level and determination are a model for other runners to aspire to. They give us something to work toward, and although we might gasp when we hear their times, there is a tiny flicker of possibility that we could someday run that fast. They give us something to reach for.

Sometimes it is the back of the pack that inspires me even more. I always think this is where the most interesting stories are. There is a variety of inspiration coming from the back, mostly coming from an individual who has overcome a challenge.

Many people slow down at a certain age and as a society this is what we expect. There are, however, older people in every race who refuse to give in to time. They run with determination, often beating people much younger than they are. These people show us what spirit and heart can do. They are not afraid to push on.

Another group who inspires me are those struggling with weight or other health issues. The people who are overweight know they are going to an event where they will see a lot of people who are in top shape. I always think these are the people who have decided to turn their life around and each step helps them become closer to the goal. I have heard stories of people who have beaten cancer, and running is a way to prove they are stronger than the illness. No matter what the issue, these are the people who struggle the most to complete the race, but they showed up and completed the task. They show determination and courage.

One man who inspired me completed an entire three-mile race with a walker. He wasn't going to allow an injury to keep him from completing a race for a cause he wanted to support.

Here is an article I wrote called "Fearless Running," which describes what inspires me.

I am a planner and someone who needs to feel prepared for everything. Because of this, whenever I have a longer race, I put a great deal of thought into my training plan, and I work as hard as I can to log as many miles as possible so that I will be ready on race day.

About a year ago, I started to notice a different type of runner. These were people who didn't let challenges or circumstances get in their way. Their attitude toward running the harder races was "Why not?" "What's the worst that could happen?" I saw women who did not fit the stereotype of the marathon runner, men and women in their eighties who knew they were going to do just as well as the twenty-year-old next to them. These are the people who don't make excuses, who don't let fear rob them of life experiences. These fearless runners are the ones who inspire me. Let me list some of the ones who have stood out.

My friend, Sally, loves to run but hadn't trained for months because of school and work. I said "Sally, want to do a half-marathon this weekend?" She didn't even hesitate before she said yes.

Maurice, the man who had to have frequent brain operations to relieve the swelling on his brain. He said that he ran because he was grateful he could.

Marcie, who had been diagnosed with brain cancer and who wanted to prove she was stronger than the disease.

Ellen, who had undergone heart surgery, and like Maurice, was grateful for her health and determined to keep it.

Marcus, who at ninety wants to prove age is only a number.

I saw a girl running a half-marathon who started to have an asthma attack, pulled out her inhaler, breathed in the medicine and kept on going.

There was a boy whose leg was injured, and each step looked painful. He just kept looking straight ahead and pushing on.

I am about to do another marathon, but this year I have had difficulty putting in the miles between work and family demands. Now, I could easily make excuses like so many do and say why I should not do the marathon, but I think it's time for me to do a little fearless running.

Have you ever felt that God put someone in front of you for a reason to inspire you? That is what I feel about Riley. Here is her story:

When I first met Riley, I was at a school retreat hiking up the side of a mountain with a group of students and teachers. The hike is famous for how difficult it is because it is a sharp incline all the way to the top.

After the first ten minutes, I came up to two girls who had stopped, and one was having difficulty breathing. I stopped to help her and the school trainer who was right behind me also stopped. We waited until her breathing was under control and I explained to her how difficult the rest of the hike was, but I told her that I would stay with her if she wanted to continue. Without hesitation she said, "I want to keep going." I knew right then that this girl had spirit, because many people would have turned around and gone back home. My friend passed us and said "Jen, this is Riley, she's a runner." I started to talk to her about running and as we stopped and rested here and there, I asked her what was causing her breathing issues. She told me that it had started about two months ago and the doctors had diagnosed her with PVM (paradoxical vocal cord dysfunction). PVM is when the vocal cords do not open correctly, and breathing is impaired. The doctors do not seem to know of a cure for PVM, and Riley has had to make some adjustments to her running routine.

Before her breathing issues, Riley was on the varsity cross country team, and she was running in the low 20 minutes for a 5k. She has had to drop down to the j.v. team and she says that she must stop in the middle of a race when her breathing becomes bad. Any runner can imagine how frustrating that would be, especially when greatness is within your grasp. Riley could be bitter, and no one would fault her but here is what she told me about her attitude. "I think this was God's way of telling me that I didn't have to be a perfect runner, that maybe I should have more fun with my running and rest a little more. Before my breathing became an issue, running was everything for me, now I know that I should just enjoy it."

Just because she has accepted that she has a serious problem does not mean she is giving up on becoming a better runner. I was talking about her to one of the football coaches when he said

"Now, I know what she was doing. I saw her running around the outside of the field and occasionally, she would stop and then start again. She kept at it for quite a while." I said to him "That's because no matter what the doctors say, she is not going to give up. Riley's not a quitter, she's a fighter."

When I asked Riley what her goals were, she told me she was just trying to get better and to take a little time off her 5k speed. When she feels her breathing becoming impaired, she knows she must stay calm and practice deep breathing techniques. It also means that she often must stop in the middle of a race to get her breathing back before she can continue.

Imagine the courage it takes to go for a run when at any moment you could be struggling to pull in enough air, but Riley is not letting her breathing issues hold her back. She has goals like any other runner, and she sees her breathing problems as an obstacle to overcome not as an excuse to give up. Riley is proof that big things come in little packages. She may be petite and slight on the outside, but she is a powerhouse when it comes to character and tenacity. Riley is an inspiration for the rest of us because, she has determination, and she shows us the possibilities within all of us.

Next time you go to a race, look around and see the variety of people. Take some time to talk to strangers and learn their stories, because everyone has one.

9   Healing the Injuries

Most runners have at least one injury during their running career. Sometimes it can be caused by overuse, a fall, a tweak, bad equipment, or an unfortunate event. It can happen to both beginners and veterans, and the longer you run the more you will know about some common injuries and how to treat them. Here are a few of the most common injuries as well as some tricks and tools that will help you with healing.

The 10% rule.

If you are wondering if you can add more miles on your weekly running total, the general rule is to not increase your mileage by more than 10%. You want to increase your mileage gradually to allow your body to adjust. If you try to do too much too soon, you will be sore, and working out consistently is better than doing too much.

Hydration

Drinking enough water is a good idea no matter what you are doing, and it is especially important if you are exercising. If you are working out for more than an hour, you also need some electrolytes. Experiment with which kind works best for you. I cannot drink Powerade or Gatorade because they are too harsh on my stomach. I found a brand called Hoist that I buy from Amazon.

Stretching

I didn't stretch very much until I turned fifty, and then my body let me know it needed some extra care. I bought a pair of shoes that were inexpensive and didn't have much support, and then I wore them exclusively for two weeks, which resulted in a neuroma. This is when nerves experience extreme compression and nerve irritation. The compression causes the nerves to swell. I was told to stretch and ice the area. At the same time, I developed plantar fasciitis, which is bottom of the heel pain. Wearing inserts, stretching, and icing can help.

Once my foot started to heal, I noticed my left leg would become stiff after a race. It gradually became worse until my hip and knee started to ache. I should have gone to have it checked, but I kept running until one day a sharp pain went through my knee and I had difficulty putting weight on it. An MRI showed I had strained my knee and I would need four weeks of physical therapy. I was disappointed I could not run, but I learned so much from the physical training about protecting myself from injury.

I was told stretching was very important. I was also told to do hip strengthening exercises and core work. Strength training is important to keep your muscles strong and injury free.

Massage

I used to think having a massage was a frill, but I now know it is an important form of self-care. Massage can improve circulation, decrease muscle stiffness, improve the quality of sleep, aid with recovery between workouts, and improve flexibility.

Rotate shoes

Shoes will last longer and serve you better if you rotate them regularly. Studies show that rotating running shoes can reduce the risk of injuries by up to 39 %, because rotating them ensures the shoes provide the cushioning and stability they should.

Cross training

Cross training is like rotating your shoes. By doing other exercises, you are using a variety of muscles instead of putting strain on the same ones every day, so you are protecting your body from injury. Other sports will still build your fitness level and help your running performance.

I had an issue with cross training for many years because I didn't feel as if I was exercising unless I ran, and I was obsessed with accumulating mileage. Injuries showed me that more isn't always better, but variety will make me a stronger runner.

Experiment with other exercises. If you go to the gym, try the elliptical, the rowing machine, and the stair stepper. In good weather, swim or walk or bike. Explore the options and have fun.

Adjust for your age

Many runners say they stopped running because of their age. They felt that running was causing too much strain on their body. You might have to adapt to how you run and how far you run, but I think running keeps your body younger. I believe in the expression, "Use it or lose it."

10   Running Heals with Hope

I mentioned earlier there was a time when I thought doing an ultra-marathon was an impossibility for me, but all I had to do was show up and start asking veteran runners questions. I made every mistake in the book, but I learned from each one. I saw that people of all fitness levels had the courage to show up. I realized the best way to change the impossible to possible was to do it! Running has shown me there is always hope you can do something that seems difficult.

Every time I do an ultra I hope I can achieve something new. Running is an activity that makes it easy to chart improvement, and with an ultra you are always hoping you can push your limits a little farther.

People who are regularly active have a stronger sense of purpose, and they experience more hope.

Running can elevate your mood and make social connections easier, and the community you can build makes you feel protected and loved, giving you hope for the future.

When we run together at a race to promote a cause, we gain a feeling of collective strength, hope, and optimism. Making a difference suddenly seems possible.

Running shows you that you can push your limits, and when you feel as if you don't have anything left, you find out you do. Running gives you hope you can do more.

Kelly McGonigal writes in *The Joy of Movement*, "If there is a voice in your head saying, "You're too old, too awkward, too big, too broken, too weak," physical sensations from movement can provide a compelling counterargument."

There is a feeling of freedom when you run. It feels as if you are in a safe space where anything can be shared without worrying about any consequences. Maybe it is because you don't have to look someone straight in the eyes, and you also don't have to look for a reaction. I have heard confessions and revelations while on long runs, and the peacefulness of nature around us helped us brainstorm solutions when they were necessary. There is hope for resolution of our problems when we are running.

Healing often starts when we reveal what is hurting us. Once we reveal it to another person, we can begin to deal with it fully and see the possibilities for healing. Most runners want to share stories and listen to the stories of others. We are all hoping we might hear those words of wisdom we need.

Running gives us hope there is something to heal us when other things we have tried have not worked. When we run, we start to see there are possibilities. We might be able to beat our illness whether it is mental or physical. Running gives us a weapon to fight against something that was overwhelming us. It can show us there is hope to find the right group of friends, to be able to interact in a healthy way with others. If we can improve with running and conquer our goals, then we can improve and conquer other challenges in life. When we can prove what our body can do, there is hope for change.

Kelly McGonigal is the author of *The Joy of Movement, How Exercise Helps Us find Happiness Hope Connection and Courage.* Kelly says, "If you are willing to move," she writes, "your muscles will give you hope. Your brain will orchestrate pleasure. And your entire physiology will adjust to help you find the energy, purpose and courage you need to keep going."

I try to run a 5k almost every weekend. A friend commented that I was spending a lot of money on races. I responded that the races helped me to stay motivated and trained, and the money was going to good causes, so I felt like I was giving back a little.

Races can bring attention to causes that need funding. One of my favorites is "Miles for Maria," which is an Ultra to bring awareness to epilepsy. The race director's daughter has epilepsy and some other medical issues. When she comes out to run a mile or two with us, it motivates us to keep going. We are running a race next week called "Backpack Buddies." The money will go toward buying school supplies for students who cannot afford them.

We run a race after Christmas to benefit a daycare for low-income children. The winners in each age group receive a pot the children have decorated with handprints, and inside the pot is a bulb that will bloom into a beautiful flower.

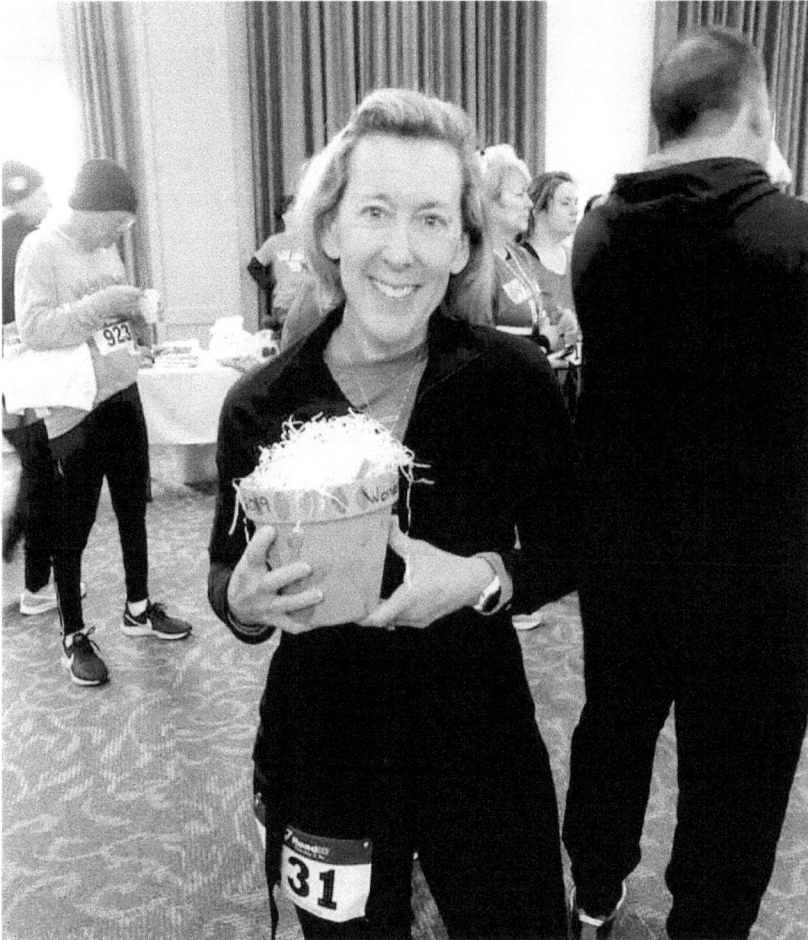

This race that benefitted a daycare handed out bulbs in pots the children had decorated.

The children are all there with their parents, and they take turns handing out their creations.

Another of my favorite runs for a cause is one that supports retired greyhounds. The organization chooses a dog that you are partnering with, and after the race you can have your picture with the dog. I am a dog lover, so it is a great morning for me to meet so many animals.

Some runs are in the memory of someone. There is a run near us called the "Tim Crunk race." Tim was passionate about running and about helping the people of Haiti. When he died, his wife decided to start a race in his name to raise money to send to help the people of Haiti.

One of my friends hosts a race to raise money for breast cancer research. The cause is special to her because several of her friends have battled breast cancer. It is nice to see the huge crowd that comes out to support the cause.

Many of the trail runs support local parks and trails. That is an important cause, because it makes these beautiful areas accessible to the community.

I am usually excited to be able support the many important causes, but one organizer made me cry before the race. The race was to fight bullying, and the organizer had brought out several children who had been bullied in school, but who had found healing through running. The running club showed them they had value and gave them an outlet for their emotions.

There is a race called "Guns n Hoses" to support police and firefighters. Members from each department interact with the community at the rac,e giving everyone a chance to get to know them better.

We run a race every year called "Run for the Son." The money raised supports the youth ministry in a local church. It is used to help youth go on mission trips to serve in the community.

Many races are a memorial to a lost loved one. It is a way for the family to remember a loved one in a positive way, and to bring awareness to a larger community. It also allows that community to wrap the family up in love. This weekend we are going to this kind of a race, called "Brees' Miles for Memory." The race remembers a young lady who loved running and her community, and Dr. Seuss. Participants are asked to dress up like a Dr. Seuss character.

"Run for Hope" is a race to benefit a women's homeless shelter. The goal is to raise money to support their mission of providing a safe and nurturing environment and supporting women to make changes in their lives.

There are races for every cause you can think of, and a race as a fundraiser is a winning situation since runners and walkers are coming out to improve both their health and their community.

Most of the races we do leave us wanting to do better. The people involved are trying to better their community. They are people of action who are determined to make a difference despite challenges they may have.

This is a winning situation because runners give to an important cause while improving their health and feeling inspired because they are part of making a difference

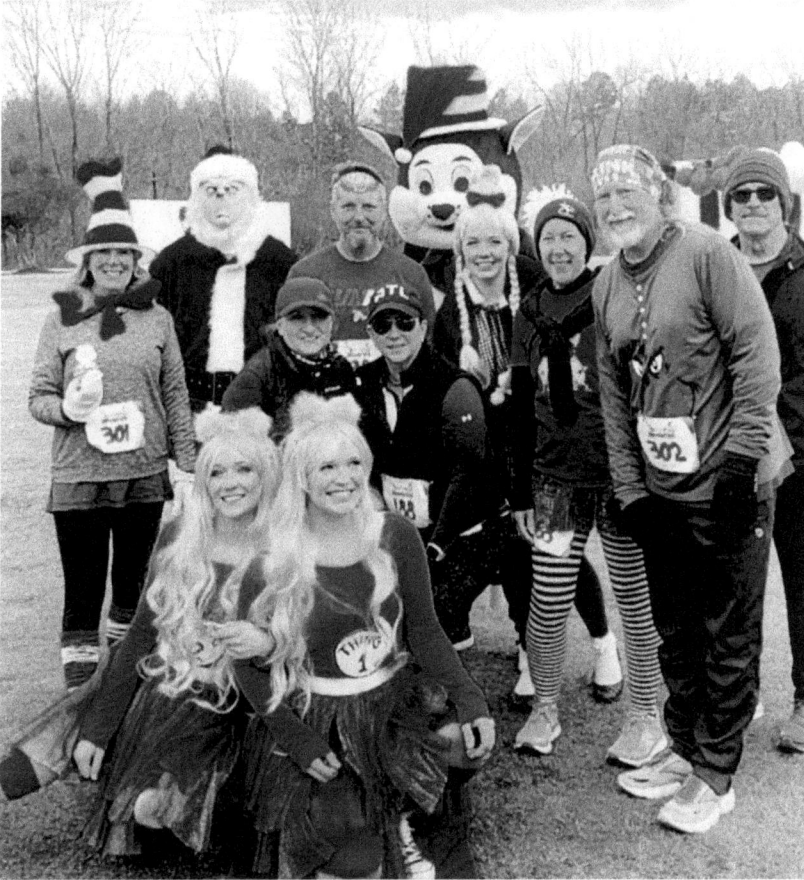

The run in memory of Bree.

11   Finding a Healthy Balance

You will often hear people ask how much they should run, and that is an answer that will vary with each individual, but too much of a good thing can cause problems instead of healing. You might think if running can make you healthy then more is better, but too much exercise can have harmful effects.

I couldn't understand why my husband was angry when I signed up for longer races, but I knew I had to tell him ahead of time to allow him to adjust to the idea. Even when I was only running a 5K, he would try to find a reason why I shouldn't go. He loves to tell me when the weather will be bad for a race, even though he knows we have run in all kinds of weather. One day I told him about a distance race, and I could see he was angry. I decided it was time to talk about this. I said, "You know how much I love to run. Why do you become so angry when I race?"

He replied, "Because I'm afraid you will hurt yourself."

That surprised me and I answered, "Honey, I'll be OK. I know my limits."

He said, "That's what I'm afraid of, because you will push right up against those limits."

We made a deal. I told him I would be careful, and I asked him if he would be my crew when I did ultras. He is now part of the experience, and we both enjoy it.

When I take a break I call him to check in and he says, "How many miles have you done? Do you

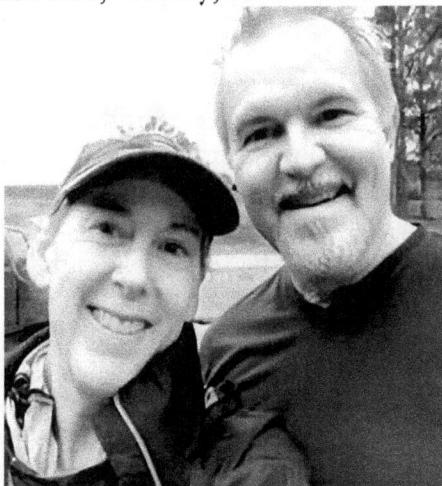

John and I at a recent ultra

need anything?"

Running can become an addiction, and it can be hard for you to realize it at first. You may start out with short runs in the neighborhood once or twice a week, but you find several months later that missing a run is disturbing to you. You feel the need to get a run in every day, you are exercising at least two hours a day, and running seems to be the center of your universe. You are missing family events because the run is more important to you, and you plan your whole day around your run. These are possible signs that running has gone from being a healing factor in your life to something that is receiving too much of your focus. My friend Michael describes it well here.

"I have been a runner for 40 years now. All those years and all those miles will forever be etched fondly in my memory, but they have also taken their toll on my body, and in some ways, my life. For years, I could not imagine taking a vacation that didn't center on a race. Kelli and I have had some great experiences with that mindset, but suddenly, it is no longer a priority.

"I have missed opportunities to watch my grandkids playing their little league games because there was a local 5K that caused a conflict. I always chose the race. I have chosen to not go out on Friday nights simply because I had to get up early for a race or a long run the next morning. But those days are over. There is more to life than running, and it is time for some of those other things to take center stage."

Michael posts about his runs every day and you can feel the positivity they cause. He runs with his wife, or heads out for a quiet, early morning jog. He is finding joy in his runs again.

There are many reasons that running can become an obsession. In the running community, many runners keep track of how many miles they run per week, and training programs often suggest a certain number of miles for success at a certain distance. There are also clubs like the 1,000-mile club which encourages runners to run 1,000 miles in a year. Runners post their times, their mileage, and their placement in the races, and although they have every right to do that and we celebrate their accomplishments, it also feeds the message that the goal is to be faster and to run longer. Most runners do this to test their limits and to chart improvements, but it is easy to be caught up in the constant push to be better. There are messages everywhere to push for more miles, but the truth is that trying to always do more might cause more harm than good. The problem with an exercise routine like this where there is no time for rest or recovery is your body will start to break down. Focusing on quality not quantity might be the answer. Give your body time to relax.

Some Signs You Might Be Overtraining.

Increased heart rate

Do you notice your heart rate is fast even when you are not running? If you are exercising too much, you could be putting extra stress on your heart. Monitor your heart rate throughout the day and compare several days throughout the week. Your heart may need a rest.

Are you always injured, sore, or ill?

If your body is being pushed too hard and doesn't have time to restore itself, it will break down in the form of injuries and sickness.

Are you always tired or have trouble sleeping?

Overuse can affect your body's daily pattern and throw off your sleep schedule. Running uses a lot of energy, so you need to give your body some time to recharge.

Are you moody?

There is a hormone called catecholamine which is related to the flight or fight hormone and overstressing the body can stir it up.

Are you always thirsty?

When your body is overstressed it is searching for restoration and that often comes in the form of dehydration. Take a sip and chill.

Gaining weight

If the body is pushed too far without enough rest, it will think there is a problem and hang on to fat.

I believe we often are sent messages through others about our wellbeing. We have to be open to hearing them, and I have been missing them completely until recently. Although running has always helped me mentally, I had gradually allowed it to consume me to the point I was neglecting many other elements of my life. The first messages I was sent were that I needed to control the amount of time devoted to running, and they came to me when I asked friends who are elite runners what they did for training. Two of them said they didn't run much during the week. They did the elliptical and raced on the weekend. I was frustrated because I was running every day and logging at least 30-40 miles a week. I decided they must be natural runners.

I also was surprised how many friends trained for races and then didn't run again until it was time for another big race. I know how painful it can be to get back into shape when you have taken too much time off, but they had the right idea to take some time to heal.

My next message came when I went with my daughter and her friends on a weekend beach vacation. I was out running when I had my first Afib attack. My pulse started racing, I couldn't catch my breath, and I felt as if I was going to pass out. I had to be taken to the hospital. When I asked the doctor what had caused the attack, he said we might never know.

After several days, I began to run excessively again until my dog collided with my shin at full speed. Several days later, my knee began to feel weak, and eventually I could barely walk on it. After an MRI, I was told I had a torn meniscus and a baker's cyst. I would like to think it was from the collision with the dog, but I think the extra miles I was running probably contributed to the problem.

When my knee started to feel better I tried to run a little. I was doing 30 minutes on the elliptical and then I would walk/run 4 miles. I was taking 2 hours out of my day to exercise.

My heart began to flutter and although it was not an Afib attack, it scared me. My trip to the cardiologist frustrated me since they wanted to put me on more medication, so I decided to try something new. I went to see an acupuncturist. After speaking with me for several minutes he said, "Jennifer, let your body heal. You're doing too much, and it's tired. Let your knee heal. Your running has become an addiction."

I'm not sure why his words penetrated my thick skull when I hadn't listened to others saying the same thing, but I am grateful I finally heard the truth. I think the extra miles made me feel as if I had accomplished something. It made me feel like an athlete. Unfortunately, my body started to break down because I was doing too much. I have recently settled on a healthy balance where running is something I do for pleasure and to calm my mind, but I now run shorter distances every other day, and I make sure to vary my exercise routine and get plenty of rest. This doesn't mean I won't be doing an ultramarathon from time to time, but the next day I will be lounging on the couch watching movies and napping. I have an even deeper peace when I run now. I appreciate every step, and I'm not concerned about how fast I am going, or how many miles I log. I will always be passionate about running, but I don't need to be consumed by it. My friend, Doug, often says to me, "More writing, less running." I use it to remind me I have other interests in my life.

I do think it is amazing I have realized my body needs to heal from running while I am writing a book about the healing power it can have. It shows there are two sides to everything, and extremes are rarely good.

If you are wondering where the line is between being passionate about running and being obsessed by it, and healed rather than hurt, I can explain it in very simple terms. I can find joy in running and be passionate about it, but I have a problem the minute it is the only focus in my life, or it is hurting other parts of my life. When my oldest wants to do something on race day, she often asks me first if I have a race that day because she thinks I will choose that over spending time with her. I am going to make sure she now knows time with family is more important. This morning, I was going to run/walk 4 miles in the neighborhood when my youngest came out on the porch and said, "Mom, want to go to Kohls?" I said yes and four miles changed to finishing up the third mile. Running will always be important to me, but I am finding a healthy balance.

Everyone will have a different idea of what a good balance is. Be aware of how you feel physically and mentally, and adjust your routine accordingly.

12   Starting Your Healing Journey

Are you ready to see what running can do for you? Here are the basics to help you get started.

Running can seem like an insurmountable task to some people. They see slender people who are scantily clad with colorful shoes racing past them and they say "Oh, no, I could never do that." Well, why not? Running is a great way to strengthen your body, lose weight, control stress, improve your mood, and with some simple steps anyone can get started. Here are some basics to get you on your way.

1. **Keep your head up and run tall with your arms at a 90-degree angle.** This allows you to breathe at maximum capacity. This is also about being relaxed as well as not wasting movement by having your arms flailing about.

2. **Keep your shoulders relaxed and focus on breathing.** It is very common for beginning runners to tense up their shoulders. This will result in painful cramping in their shoulders. Run with your body completely relaxed. This will also help to avoid some injuries since, a loose body reacts to certain situations better than a tense, rigid one. New runners will sometimes hold their breath because they are so focused on running. Focus on regular breathing in and out until it becomes second nature.

3. **Never run through an injury.** A small problem can become a larger one if it is ignored. It is often difficult for a runner to take time off, but a little rest can prevent the need to be sidelined for longer periods.

4. **Feet should follow a straight line.** This will help to keep your body aligned. Runners who point their feet to their sides often end up with hip and knee problems.

5. Lean into hills with short strides and control running downhill. Shortening your stride and leaning into the hill will make it easier to get up it faster. Hill running also requires some mental training. Remember, it is only a hill. Have some mental boosters ready to repeat as you ascend. An example would be "I will not stop, you cannot defeat me, I will conquer this." It is surprising how well this works. When going downhill, control the way your feet impact the ground. Many runners slam their feet down with each step and end up with shin splints. Lean forward into the hill and run through it.

6. Do a variety of different types of runs. Do some long slow runs because you have to build a base of miles in order to run well. A long slow run is also a great way to ease out the kinks and unwind. We say we are doing LSD (long slow distance) the runner's drug. Run some hills. Hill running not only makes you faster and stronger, but also helps you with technique. It also prepares you mentally for a hilly course. Do some speedwork, because the only way to get faster is to run faster. Speedwork is also a great way to learn how to pace yourself.

7. Run softly. Pay attention to how hard your feet hit the ground. If you can lessen the impact when you run, you have less chance of injury.

8. Buy good shoes and take care of your feet. Everything starts with shoes. They can protect you from injury, so find a good pair. Pay attention to what is happening to your feet. Apply lotion after running to make sure they do not crack. Check for blisters and black toes.

9. Drink plenty of fluids and eat a variety of food. Most of us do not drink enough fluid even when we are not exercising, and a deficiency of fluids can make us sluggish. When we are running, we lose fluids and need to replace them. The best way to avoid dehydration is to drink a little all day. You know you are drinking enough if when you go to the bathroom your urine is clear. Do not follow the fad of the day whether it is a high protein or low carbohydrates. Eat a variety of healthy foods.

10. Understand the mental aspect of running. Several things will benefit you mentally. You have to be confident you will do your best. You have to work on a positive attitude and practice positive self-talk. Play games when you run like counting how many runners you pass. Never go out with a defeatist attitude. It will slow you down much faster than shin splints. Set goals and decide how you will meet them.

Goals

What would you like to achieve in the future and what can you shoot for in the short term? An example would be that you want to complete a marathon by the end of the year, and to do that you are going to gradually do longer races until you feel you are ready for the marathon.

- Investing time in training: Spend some time planning your training. Make it enjoyable and vary your routines. You have to put in the time to see the results.

- Trail running: Go off-road and try some trail running. You will see beautiful views and have a different set of challenges from road running.

- Attitude: Be your number one fan and celebrate the successes. Believe you can achieve anything you attempt.

- Never giving up: Try not to give in to frustration. Everyone has days when they want to run farther than their body wants to, there will be days when it is better to take a day off.

- Extra miles: If you want to be a distance runner, you have to run distance. Set aside some time to fit in some extra runs.

Running Gear

Good Shoes

I know we are going through a minimalist phase right now and barefoot running is still popular, but I know I personally need a good pair of shoes. When I coached running, I found that most injuries stemmed from a problem with the shoes. Go to a running store and have someone evaluate your running style. Ask their advice about the shoe you need to match your style and mileage. If you can afford two pairs, it is a good idea to switch them out and wear them on alternate days. I learned I had to buy a half a size bigger than I needed for a street shoe. Spending money on a good pair of shoes could eliminate the aggravation of an injury later.

A foam roller

This is a round piece of foam that is used to roll out aches and pains. They can be found at most stores including Wal-Mart and Target. Position the roller under the aching muscle and roll back and forth on top of it. It is fairly painful but a great way to help your muscles recover.

The stick

This is used for the same thing as the roller, but it is easier to use. It looks like a long baton, and you just run it over the muscles.

A tennis ball.

This can be used for the same things as the stick and the roller, but it is more portable. It works great on sore shoulders too.

Elastic bands/resistance bands

You can buy pieces of elastic and use them to strengthen your legs. Put them around your feet and do leg lifts. You can also use them for arm exercises. You can also use resistance bands to stretch.

Compression socks/sleeves

Compression socks and sleeves can aid in recovery, and they are also helpful during running. You can also find sleeves for things like sore it bands.

Balance board

Balance is an important health component and balance boards can be fun. Once you think you can keep the board steady, add something to it like bouncing a tennis ball off the wall and catching it while keeping your balance. You can buy them at almost all department stores or running stores.

Epsom salts

These are placed in the bath to help soothe sore muscles.

A hat for rainy runs

Rainy runs can be beautiful, but you need something to keep the water out of your eyes, so a baseball cap is a necessity in the toolbox.

Fuel

If you are doing a high intensity or long run it's a good idea to carry something to eat with you. You can choose from a variety of bars, energy waffles or gels. Find what you enjoy.

Pepto Bismol tablets especially on long runs

Runners occasionally have gastrointestinal distress, especially on long rungs and Pepto Bismol tablets can avoid a painful situation.

Comfy running clothes

Running clothes do not have to be expensive. I have found my favorite running clothes at the local thrift store. Wear what you are comfortable in. Experiment with different fabrics and different layers during colder weather. Do not experiment with anything the day of a race though. It's best to go with tried and true on those days.

Vaseline

Running stores sell body glide that helps avoid chafing but Vaseline works just as well and it's less expensive.

Bio freeze

You will eventually experience sore muscles. Bio freeze can help keep you comfortable.

Weights

Weights can help strengthen your muscles to prevent injuries.

Inspiration

Inspiration can be found in readings that motivate you, a friend who supports you, or a fellow runner who runs despite a disability or hardship. All you have to do to find this type of inspiration is go to a race and be an observer.

A running log

Track your progress by writing down your workouts and how you felt. Record races and times and plan your goals.

A little dash of crazy

This comes in handy when your friend convinces you to run a race that requires training that you have not done, or when the weather is horrific, or you are asked to run in a race that involves zombies chasing you, obstacles, or great quantities of mud.

If you can have at least some of these items in your possession, your adventure with running will probably go smoother.

The ABCs of Running

Most of the time, reducing wisdom to its most basic form gives us the greatest benefit. An example of this would be to look at running advice in the form of the ABC.

Add more mileage gradually. 10% more per week is the recommended amount.

Be a cheerleader for yourself. Celebrate the triumphs and don't worry too much about the rest.

Continue to try to improve.

Decide what your challenge is going to be and get ready to meet it.

Energize with nutritious food.

Forget all your problems and enjoy a great run.

Get a good playlist on your iPod.

Hydrate.

Invest in a good pair of shoes. Many injuries stem from poor shoes. Protect yourself.

Just run and have fun.

Keep track of your time and your mileage.

Love your feet. They are carrying you and they need tender care.

Mentally prepare yourself to run.

Never run through an injury.

Openly recruit friends to run with you.

Prepare for a race.

Question veteran runners to find what works for them.

Rest.

Set goals.

Try new routes and routines.

Understand that there will be days your body does not want to run.

Value a good long run.

Weather is not always an excuse not to run. Dress accordingly.

X out injuries with common sense.

Yell for and encourage others in your races.

Zeal will keep you going when your body does not want to.

13   Crossing the Finish Line

Writing this book was an act of love. Running has meant so much to me and it has been such a gift. I hope that readers will see the possibilities of what running can do in their own lives. Running can offer a different type of healing for everyone. You might need to use it as an escape so you can have some peace and quiet and not need to talk to anyone but yourself.

When I was teaching, there were students calling my name nonstop. They needed me to help, and I was glad to do it, but I often felt as if I was being pulled in a million different directions. It is hard to think when someone is always asking for your attention. When I went for a run I had the quiet I needed to refocus, and problem solve. Some days I could let my body and mind unwind as the miles slipped past.

Some let running become their power against a disease or a situation. If you are strong enough to run, you are strong enough to survive illness, or a difficult situation. The negatives do not define you when you can use the positive aspects of running to give you hope.

Running can heal you by giving you a connection to a community. That community might be your friends, a running club, or the people you meet at races. One of my connections is with my neighborhood. I run in our subdivision because it is safe, and I don't have to watch out for cars. It gives me a chance to stop and talk with neighbors, and it never gets old when the neighborhood children yell from the porch, "Hey, Miss Jen!"

You can be healed spiritually with running because it allows you to be out in nature while you listen to what's happening around you. You can take in all the beauty and reflect on the glory of nature.

Deep breathing is a healthy technique we all can benefit from doing. While you are running, practice taking a deep breath in, hold it, and then release it slowly.

Running will allow you to run away from those things that feel like they are crushing you. It is a healthy escape where you can release all your emotions as you move forward toward something better.

As you run more and you see the improvements running can give you, you also realize you can make those changes in other parts of your life. It gives you hope.

Running will always be my reaction when I am overwhelmed. If I am hurt, unsettled, perplexed, or full of joy I feel better when I head out for a run. It feels as if I am turning my energy in the right direction. I also have a feeling I am taking steps toward fixing something that might be too much for me emotionally. Sitting still and being swamped by all the feelings can make things worse, but if I can head off down the road as if I am chasing answers I can tell myself I am moving toward resolution.

I would love to show people that running is not a one-size-fits-all sport. It can be adjusted to fit what you need and what you are comfortable with doing. If you want to, go out and walk and run for a half hour, or train for a race. Anything goes. Don't allow the fear of not fitting in, or not being good enough keep you from trying a sport that can change your life. Take that first step out of your comfort zone, and whether you do it by yourself or you convince a friend to join you, give running a chance.

I will end with another quote from Scott Jurek's his book, *Eat And Run: My Unlikely Journey to Ultramarathon Greatness.*

> A 100-mile race or a 5K, or a run around the block won't cure pain, but you can be transformed. Not overnight, but over time. Life is not a race. There is no finish line. We strive toward a goal, and whether we achieve it or not is important, but it's not what's most important. What matters is how we move toward that goal. (p. 227)

In my opinion, running can help you reach those goals and keep you healthy mentally and physically on your way.

Bibliography

Brown, J. (2015). *The runner's brain*. Workman Publishing.

Ellis, J. (2013). *Running injury-free: How to prevent, treat, and recover from runner's knee, shin splints, sore feet, and every other ache and pain*. Rodale.

Fixx, J. F. (2018). *The Complete Book of Running*. Ishi Press International.

Hall, R. (2019). *Run the mile you're in: Finding god in every step*. Zondervan.

Jurek, S., & Friedman, S. (2013). *Eat & Run: My unlikely journey to ultramarathon greatness*. Mariner Books.

Kerr Kalin, K. K. (2021, October 10). *A&M to highlight addiction recovery in 5K run*. The Battalion. Retrieved March 29, 2023, from https://www.thebatt.com/news/a-m-to-highlight-addiction-recovery-in-5k-run/article_b3639036-2a1e-11ec-9196-7f1d30b948e9.html.

Koop, J., Rutberg, J., & Malcolm, C. (2021). *Training essentials for ultrarunning*. Koop Endurance Services.

Laneve, N. (2022, May 3). *6 benefits of exercise in addiction recovery: Potential treatment for drug abuse*. The Recovery Village Drug and Alcohol Rehab. Retrieved March 29, 2023, from https://www.therecoveryvillage.com/recovery/wellness/6-proven-benefits-exercise-addiction-recovery/.

Marandi-Steves, Sarah. (2019, May 18). *How running heals the mind, body, and soul*. Sarah Marandi-Steeves, LCSW, PLLC. Retrieved March 30, 2023, from

https://smsteevesblog.com/2018/07/14/how-running-heals-the-mind-body-and-soul/.

Martin Ginis, K. (n.d.). *How can exercise improve body image?* Medical News Today. Retrieved March 30, 2023, from https://www.medicalnewstoday.com/articles/317958.

McGonigal, K. (2021). *The joy of movement: How exercise helps us find happiness, hope, connection, and courage.* Avery, an imprint of Penguin Random House LLC.

Newkey-Burden, C. (2021). *The little book of running: For everyone from the beginner to the long-distance runner.* OH!

Rasa, C. (2020, January 16). *Why running is good for addiction recovery.* Podium Runner. Retrieved March 29, 2023, from https://www.podiumrunner.com/culture/running-good-addicts-recovery/.

Ratey, J. (2022, July 7). *The effects of exercise on the brain with dr. John Ratey.* KineSophy. Retrieved March 29, 2023, from https://kinesophy.com/the-effects-of-exercise-on-the-brain-with-dr-john-ratey/.

Volkow, N. (2008, June 9). *Working out may help prevent substance abuse.* NBCNews.com. Retrieved March 29, 2023, from https://www.nbcnews.com/health/health-news/working-out-may-help-prevent-substance-abuse-flna1C9453107.

Weingus, L. (2022, September 23). *7 reasons running improves confidence.* mindbodygreen. Retrieved March 30, 2023, from https://www.mindbodygreen.com/articles/why-running-improves-confidence.

What you can learn from Jeff Galloway's 40-plus years of running. Runner's World. (2021, November 2). Retrieved March 30, 2023, from https://www.runnersworld.com/runners-stories/a22997370/jeff-galloway-interview/.

Wiginton, K. (2021, May 11). *Exercise: How It Can Help With Addiction Recovery.* WebMD. Retrieved March 29, 2023, from https://www.webmd.com/mental-health/addiction/

exercise-help-addiction-recovery.

About the Author

Running for Jennifer Bonn has always been more than exercise. She sees it as something that can help us mentally, physically, spiritually, and socially. Jennifer has always been active in sports, but in college she began to see the benefits of running beyond merely conditioning. She has been an avid runner for 45 years.

Jennifer was a cross-country coach for nine years, and an assistant track coach for one. She enjoys helping others find joy in running. Jennifer runs competitively almost every weekend, and her favorite distance is the ultra-marathon, (anything over 26.2). She has written about running for *Trail Runner*, *The Running Journal*, *The Cross-Country Journal*, and she had a regular column in *Georgia Runner* called On The Run.

One of the things Jennifer loves the most is the social aspect of running. Connections are easy to make at races, and runner's stories are inspirational.

Jennifer has written several other books including *101 Tips to Lighten Your Burden: Practical Advice for Life*, and *What I Hope for You: A Grandmother's Wishes*. You can read more of her writing on her blog at www.jenniferswriting.org.

Jennifer says that running and writing are two things she loves to do because they both keep her sane and happy and she is smiling while doing them. Writing allows her to express herself and share with others while running clears her brain and allows creativity to enter.

Jennifer lives with her husband and youngest daughter in Georgia. She has three children, three grandchildren, a cat, and a border collie.

We all have burdens of some kind, though we may carry them in different ways. The way we react to our challenges in life will determine whether we continue to struggle or whether we live life to the fullest.

When we are faced with road-blocks in life, we always have choices. We can let them paralyze us and not move forward, we can bust through them leaving havoc in our wake, or we can find a way around them continuing down our path.

101 Tips to Lighten Your Burden gives you quick, easy-to-read advice on how to handle many of life's struggles. You can pick it up whenever you need a lift. It will be like the voice of a friend telling you what you can do to make the situation better.

Readers will....

- Discover ways to cope with difficult situations.
- Realize that they are not alone with what they face in life.
- Find solace in the messages given.
- See they have power to make choices by how they react.
- Feel empowered by the messages.

"I have a Ph.D. in psychology, and decades of therapeutic experience, and I can tell you, this book could have been written by an experienced psychologist. Ms. Bonn could change professions, and become a professor in the psychology department of any university. In particular, she is an expert in Positive Psychology."

--Bob Rich, PhD, *Author of From Depression to Contentment*

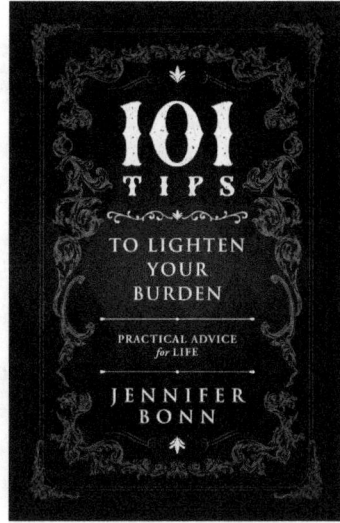

From Loving Healing Press

ISBN 978-1-61599-609-4

What I Hope for You is the story of a grandmother's life hopes for her grandchild: a combination of wishes for happiness, strong character and a life of excitement, blessings and an everyday feeling of magic.

"*What I Hope for You* perfectly captures the joy and dreams of a grandmother for her young grandchild. Jen Bonn simply, vividly and sincerely expresses the hopes and wishes many of us have for our own grandchildren to become strong, loving and fulfilled in life. I will read this book many, many times to my own young grandson."

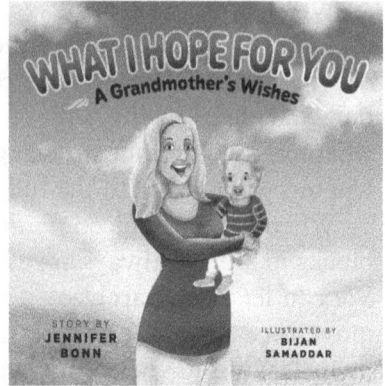

-- Donna Wood, English teacher

"*What I Hope for You* is a lovely book of a grandparent's prayer for her grandchild's future. It is filled with beautiful imagery of castles by lakes and meadows full of flowers. The author dreams of the child being around nature and sensing God's beauty in the world, but also of the child growing into an adult with beauty inside their heart."

-- Kathy Bridges, librarian

"I cannot say enough about *What I Hope for You*! I read it to my kids, and they loved it! It opened doors for wonderful questions and conversations. It is long enough to create a meaningful memory yet short enough to hold their attention. What wonderful affirmations to speak and pray over the ones we love the most!"

-- Amber Faye Wardlaw, mother of three

"As a grandmother of three, this book resonated with me, and it is exactly what I would wish for my grandchildren. The first time I read *What I Hope for You*, I remembered my time with my grandmother, and I realized that these were all wishes she had for me."

--Kimberly Tucker, aircraft mechanic III-Gen-Mods

From Loving Healing Press

ISBN 978-1-61599-739-8